W9-BNL-448

UNDERGROUND
CLINICAL VIGNETTES

. . . .

PATHOPHYSIOLOGY VOL. I

Classic Clinical Cases for
USMLE Step 1 Review [102 cases, 2nd ed]

VIKAS BHUSHAN, MD
University of California, San Francisco, Class of 1991
Series Editor, Diagnostic Radiologist

CHIRAG AMIN, MD
University of Miami, Class of 1996
Orlando Regional Medical Center, Resident in Orthopaedic Surgery

TAO LE, MD
University of California, San Francisco, Class of 1996
Yale-New Haven Hospital, Resident in Internal Medicine

VISHAL PALL, MBBS
Government Medical College, Chandigarh, India, Class of 1996

HOANG NGUYEN
Northwestern University, Class of 2000

JOSE M. FIERRO, MD
La Salle University, Mexico City
Brookdale University Hospital, New York, Intern in Medicine/Pediatrics

VIPAL SONI
UCLA School of Medicine, Class of 1999

©1999 by S2S Medical Publishing

NOTICE: The authors of this volume have taken care that the information contained herein is accurate and compatible with the standards generally accepted at the time of publication. Nevertheless, it is difficult to ensure that all the information given is entirely accurate for all circumstances. The publisher and authors do not guarantee the contents of this book and disclaim any liability, loss, or damage incurred as a consequence, directly or indirectly, of the use and application of any of the contents of this volume.

Distributed by Blackwell Science, Inc.
Editorial Office:
Commerce Place, 350 Main Street, Malden, Massachusetts 02148, USA

Distributors

USA

    Blackwell Science, Inc.
    Commerce Place
    350 Main Street
    Malden, Massachusetts 02148
    (Telephone orders: 800-215-1000 or
    781-388-8250;
    fax orders: 781-388-8270)

Canada

    Login Brothers Book Company
    324 Saulteaux Crescent
    Winnipeg, Manitoba, R3J 3T2
    (Telephone orders: 204-224-4068;
    Telephone: 800-665-1148; fax: 800-
    665-0103)

Australia

    Blackwell Science Pty, Ltd.
    54 University Street
    Carlton, Victoria 3053
    (Telephone orders: 03-9347-0300;
    fax orders: 03-9349-3016)

Outside North America and Australia

    Blackwell Science, Ltd.
    c/o Marston Book Services, Ltd.
    P.O. Box 269
    Abingdon
    Oxon OX14 4YN
    England
    (Telephone orders: 44-01235-465500;
    fax orders: 44-01235-465555)

ISBN: 1-890061-17-4

Editor: Andrea Fellows
Typesetter: Vikas Bhushan using MS Word97
Printed and bound by Capital City Press

Printed in the United States of America
99 00 01 02 6 5 4 3

All rights reserved. No part of this book may be reproduced in any form or by any electronic or mechanical means, including information storage and retrieval systems, without permission in writing from the publisher, except by a reviewer who may quote brief passages in a review.

Contributors

SAMIR MEHTA
Temple University, Class of 2000

ALEA EUSEBIO
UCLA School of Medicine, Class of 2000

MARK TANAKA
UCSF School of Medicine, Class of 1999

RICHA VARMA
Cambridge Overseas Medical Training Programme, Class of 2001

DIEGO RUIZ
UCSF School of Medicine, Class of 1999

Acknowledgments

· ·

Throughout the production of this book, we have had the support of many friends and colleagues. Special thanks to our business manager, Gianni Le Nguyen. For expert computer support, Tarun Mathur and Alex Grimm. For design suggestions, Sonia Santos and Elizabeth Sanders.

For editing, proofreading, and assistance across the vignette series, we collectively thank Carolyn Alexander, Henry E. Aryan, Natalie Barteneva, Sanjay Bindra, Julianne Brown, Hebert Chen, Arnold Chin, Yoon Cho, Karekin R. Cunningham, A. Sean Dalley, Sunit Das, Ryan Armando Dave, Robert DeMello, David Donson, Alea Eusebio, Priscilla A. Frase, Anil Gehi, Parul Goyal, Alex Grimm, Tim Jackson, Sundar Jayaraman, Aarchan Joshi, Rajni K. Jutla, Faiyaz Kapadi, Aaron S. Kesselheim, Sana Khan, Andrew Pin-wei Ko, Warren S. Krackov, Benjamin H.S. Lau, Scott Lee, Warren Levinson, Eric Ley, Ken Lin, Samir Mehta, Gil Melmed, Joe Messina, Vivek Nandkarni, Deanna Nobleza, Darin T. Okuda, Adam L. Palance, Sonny Patel, Ricardo Pietrobon, Riva L. Rahl, Aashita Randeria, Marilou Reyes, Diego Ruiz, Anthony Russell, Sanjay Sahgal, Sonal Shah, John Stulak, Lillian Su, Julie Sundaram, Rita Suri, Richa Varma, Amy Williams, Ashraf Zaman and David Zipf. Please let us know if your name has been missed or mispelled and we will be happy to make the change in the next edition.

Table of Contents

. . . .

CASE	SUBSPECIALTY	NAME
40	Gastroenterology	Achalasia
41	Gastroenterology	Acute Cholecystitis
42	Gastroenterology	Acute Hemorrhagic Gastritis
43	Gastroenterology	Acute Intestinal Obstruction
44	Gastroenterology	Acute Pancreatitis
45	Gastroenterology	Adenomatous Polyps of the Colon
46	Gastroenterology	Alcoholism
47	Gastroenterology	Appendicitis
48	Gastroenterology	Candida Esophagitis
49	Gastroenterology	Carcinoid Syndrome
50	Gastroenterology	Cecal Carcinoma
51	Gastroenterology	Celiac Disease
52	Gastroenterology	Chronic Pancreatitis
53	Gastroenterology	Diverticulitis
54	Gastroenterology	Esophageal Carcinoma
55	Gastroenterology	Esophageal Variceal Bleeding
56	Gastroenterology	Gastric Carcinoma
57	Gastroenterology	Gastric Leiomyoma
58	Gastroenterology	Gastroesophageal Reflux Disease (GERD)
59	Gastroenterology	Hemochromatosis
60	Gastroenterology	Hepatic Cirrhosis
61	Gastroenterology	Hepatocellular Carcinoma
62	Gastroenterology	Hepatorenal Syndrome
63	Gastroenterology	Intussusception
64	Gastroenterology	Ischemic Bowel Disease
65	Gastroenterology	Metastatic Carcinoma of the Liver
66	Gastroenterology	Pancreatic Carcinoma
67	Gastroenterology	Peutz–Jegher's Syndrome
68	Gastroenterology	Plummer–Vinson Syndrome
69	Gastroenterology	Posterior Duodenal Ulcer
70	Gastroenterology	Primary Biliary Cirrhosis
71	Gastroenterology	Thrombosed External Hemorrhoid
72	Gastroenterology	Wilson's Disease
73	Gastroenterology	Zollinger–Ellison Syndrome
74	Heme/Onc	Acute Hemolytic Transfusion Reaction
75	Heme/Onc	Acute Lymphoblastic Leukemia (ALL)
76	Heme/Onc	Acute Myelogenous Leukemia (AML)
77	Heme/Onc	Aplastic Anemia
78	Heme/Onc	Autoimmune Hemolytic Anemia
79	Heme/Onc	Burkitt's Lymphoma
80	Heme/Onc	Chronic Lymphocytic Leukemia (CLL)
81	Heme/Onc	Chronic Myelogenous Leukemia (CML)
82	Heme/Onc	Disseminated Intravascular Coagulation
83	Heme/Onc	Febrile Nonhemolytic Transfusion Reaction
84	Heme/Onc	Graft-versus-Host Disease (GVHD)
85	Heme/Onc	Hairy Cell Leukemia
86	Heme/Onc	Hemolytic–Uremic Syndrome
87	Heme/Onc	Henoch–Schönlein Purpura

Preface to the Second Edition

. . . .

We are very pleased with the overwhelmingly positive reception of the first edition of our *Underground Clinical Vignettes* series. In the second editions we have fine-tuned nearly every case by incorporating corrections, enhancements and clarifications. These were based on feedback from the several thousand students who used the first editions.

We implemented two structural changes upon the request of many students:

♦ bi-directional cross-linking to appropriate High Yield Facts in the 1999 edition of *First Aid for the USMLE Step 1* (Appleton & Lange);

♦ case names have been moved to the bottom of the page and obvious references to the case name within the case description have been removed.

With this, we hope they'll emerge as a unique and well-integrated study tool that provides compact clinical correlations to basic science information.

We invite your corrections and suggestions for the next edition of this book. For the first submission of each factual correction or new vignette, you will receive a personal acknowledgement and a free copy of the revised book. We prefer that you submit corrections or suggestions via electronic mail to vbhushan@aol.com. Please include "Underground Vignettes" as the subject of your message. If you do not have access to e-mail, use the following mailing address: S2S Medical Publishing, 1015 Gayley Ave, Box 1113, Los Angeles, CA 90024 USA.

Preface to the First Edition

. . . .

This series was developed to address the increasing number of clinical vignette questions on the USMLE Step 1 and Step 2. It is designed to supplement and complement *First Aid for the USMLE Step 1* (Appleton & Lange).

Each book uses a series of approximately 100 "**supra-prototypical**" **cases as a way to condense testable facts and associations.** The clinical vignettes in this series are designed to incorporate as many testable facts as possible into a cohesive and memorable clinical picture. The vignettes represent composites drawn from general and specialty textbooks, reference books, thousands of USMLE style questions and the personal experience of the authors and reviewers.

Although each case tends to present all the signs, symptoms, and diagnostic findings for a particular illness, **patients generally will not present with such a "complete" picture either clinically or on the Step 1 exam.** Cases are not meant to simulate a potential real patient or an exam vignette. All the **boldfaced "buzzwords" are for learning purposes** and are not necessarily expected to be found in any one patient with the disease.

Definitions of selected important terms are placed within the vignettes in (= SMALL CAPS) in parentheses. Other parenthetical remarks often refer to the pathophysiology or mechanism of disease. The format should also help students learn to present cases succinctly during oral "bullet" presentations on clinical rotations. The cases are meant to be read as a condensed review, not as a primary reference.

The information provided in this book has been prepared with a great deal of thought and careful research. This book should not, however, be considered as your sole source of information. Corrections, suggestions and submissions of new cases are encouraged and will be acknowledged and incorporated in future editions.

Abbreviations

. . . .

ABGs – arterial blood gases
ACE – angiotensin-converting enzyme
ACTH – adrenocorticotropic hormone
AIDS – acquired immunodeficiency syndrome
ALT – alanine transaminase
Angio – angiography
AST – aspartate transaminase
ATG – rabbit antihuman thymocyte globulin
AV - arteriovenous
BE – barium enema
BUN – blood urea nitrogen
CABG – coronary artery bypass graft
CALLA – common acute lymphoblastic leukemia antigen
CBC – complete blood count
CEA – carcinoembryonic antigen
CHF – congestive heart failure
CK – creatine kinase
COPD – chronic obstructive pulmonary disease
CT – computerized tomography
CXR – chest x-ray
DIC – disseminated intravascular coagulation
DTs – delirium tremens
ECG – electrocardiography
Echo - echocardiography
EEG – electroencephalography
EGD – esophagogastroduodenoscopy
ELISA – enzyme-linked immunosorbent assay
EMG – electromyography
ERCP – endoscopic retrograde cholangiopancreatography
ESR – erythrocyte sedimentation rate
FNA – fine needle aspiration
FSH – follicle-stimulating hormone
GERD – gastroesophageal reflux disease
GI – gastrointestinal
GnRH – gonadotropin-releasing hormone
GVHD – graft-versus-host disease
Hb - hemoglobin
HBsAg – hepatitis B surface antigen
Hct - hematocrit
HDL – high-density lipoprotein
5-HIAA – 5-hydroxyindoleacetic acid
HIDA – hepatoiminodiacetic acid [scan]
HIV – human immunodeficiency virus
HPI – history of present illness
ICU – intensive care unit
ID/CC – identification and chief complaint
IDDM – insulin-dependent diabetes mellitus
Ig – immunoglobulin
IHSS – idiopathic hypertrophic subaortic stenosis

Abbreviations - continued

IVP – intravenous pyelography
KUB – kidneys/ureter/bladder
LDH – lactate dehydrogenase
LDL – low-density lipoprotein
LH – luteinizing hormone
LP – lumbar puncture
LVH – left ventricular hypertrophy
Lytes – electrolytes
Mammo – mammography
MR – magnetic resonance [imaging]
NSAID – nonsteroidal anti-inflammatory drug
Nuc – nuclear medicine
PA – posteroanterior
PAS – periodic acid-Schiff
PBS – peripheral blood smear
PCO_2 – partial pressure of carbon dioxide
PDGF – platelet-derived growth factor
PE – physical exam
PET – positron emission tomography
PFTs – pulmonary function tests
PMN – polymorphonuclear leukocyte
PO_2 – partial pressure of oxygen
PT – prothrombin time
PTCA – percutaneous transluminal coronary angioplasty
PTT – partial thromboplastin time
RAIU – radioactive iodine uptake
RBC – red blood cell
SBFT – small bowel follow-through [barium study]
SGOT – serum glutamic-oxaloacetic transaminase
SMX-TMP – sulfamethoxazole–trimethoprim
TDT – terminal deoxytransferase
TIA – transient ischemic attack
tPA – tissue plasminogen activator
TRAP – tartrate-resistant acid phosphatase
TSH – thyroid-stimulating hormone
TTP – thrombotic thrombocytopenic purpura
UA – urinalysis
UGI – upper GI [barium study]
US – ultrasound
V/Q – ventilation perfusion
VS – vital signs
vWF – von Willebrand's factor
WBC – white blood cell
XR – x-ray

ID/CC	An asymptomatic **60-year-old** white **male** undergoing a routine physical exam is discovered to have a **pulsating abdominal mass.**
HPI	The patient has a history of **occasional abdominal pain** and **hypercholesterolemia** that has been poorly controlled by diet and medication.
PE	**Pulsating, painless upper abdominal mass** approximately 5 cm in diameter.
Labs	N/A
Imaging	KUB-Lateral: calcification of aneurysm wall. CT/US-Abdomen: dilated aorta with irregular calcified wall; large, eccentric mural thrombus seen.
Gross Pathology	Most aneurysms are located between renal arteries and iliac bifurcation; thrombus may also be present; intramural dissection may also be seen.
Micro Pathology	Aneurysm wall contains all three (intima, media, adventitia) layers (= "TRUE" ANEURYSM).
Treatment	**Surgical replacement with graft** (if > 5 cm or symptomatic); consider endovascular stent/graft.
Discussion	The risk of rupture with potentially fatal bleeding increases with size. Usually caused by **atherosclerotic** disease and often associated with coronary artery disease. Also caused by trauma, infection (e.g., syphilis), and arteritis. Sequelae include rupture, embolization, infection, and vascular occlusion secondary to thrombus formation.

. . . .

ABDOMINAL AORTIC ANEURYSM

ID/CC	A 48-year-old **male** with a history of **hypertension** is brought by ambulance to the emergency room because of the development of **sudden sharp, tearing, intractable left chest pain with radiation to the back.**
HPI	When he first arrives, he shows a declining level of consciousness, becomes **pale** and **short of breath** (= DYSPNEA), has **decreased urine output** (= OLIGURIA), and is unable to move his left arm and leg; subsequently he **faints** (= SYNCOPE).
PE	VS: **marked hypotension** (BP 90/50) in left arm, with significantly higher reading in right arm (BP 170/80). PE: **pallor; cyanosis; diaphoresis;** indistinct heart sounds; **aortic regurgitation murmur** (high-pitched, blowing, diastolic decrescendo murmur); inspiratory crackles at lung bases bilaterally (due to pulmonary edema); **anuria** (due to decreased renal perfusion); **left-sided hemiplegia.**
Labs	ECG: no evidence of myocardial infarct.
Imaging	CT/MR: **spiraling intimal flap with true and false lumen** (= DOUBLE-BARREL AORTA). Angio-Aortography: confirmatory. CXR: **mediastinal widening** (due to hemorrhage).
Gross Pathology	Longitudinal separation of tunica media of aortic wall.
Micro Pathology	N/A
Treatment	ICU monitoring for shock; antihypertensive agents to decrease vascular shear forces (avoid arteriolar dilators such as hydralazine); surgical correction.
Discussion	A **life-threatening** condition requiring immediate treatment. Predisposing factors include **hypertension** and connective tissue diseases (cystic medial necrosis as in Marfan's syndrome); complications include rupture and extension. **Sudden death** may occur with **pericardial tamponade** or **extension of dissection into coronary arteries.**

AORTIC DISSECTION

ID/CC	A 31-year-old white male who was diagnosed with **Marfan's syndrome** more than 20 years ago **recently** developed **severe shortness of breath**.
HPI	He denies smoking or drinking and claims to have had no major illnesses in the past.
PE	VS: **pulse bounding, large in volume, and collapsing** (= WATER-HAMMER OR CORRIGAN'S PULSE), producing **wide pulse pressure** with rapid rise and fall. PE: soft, high-pitched, blowing **diastolic decrescendo murmur heard best at left sternal border** with patient leaning forward and in expiration; diastolic murmur heard when femoral artery compressed with stethoscope (= DUROZIEZ' SIGN).
Labs	ECG: left ventricular hypertrophy (LVH).
Imaging	CXR: left ventricular dilatation. Echo: LVH, doppler confirmatory.
Gross Pathology	Caused by defect of aortic valves or roots that leads to regurgitation of blood from aorta into left ventricle.
Micro Pathology	N/A
Treatment	Surgical **prosthetic valve replacement**; antibiotic prophylaxis against infective endocarditis before undergoing surgical or dental procedures.
Discussion	Common causes include congenital bicuspid valve, infective endocarditis, and hypertension; less common causes include rheumatic heart disease and aortic root diseases (e.g., Marfan's syndrome, ankylosing spondylitis, Reiter's syndrome, tertiary syphilis).

. . . .

AORTIC INSUFFICIENCY

ID/CC	A **24-year-old** man complains of easy fatigability, dyspnea on mild exertion, and **angina.**
HPI	He also admits to having occasional spells of **lightheadedness** and **fainting** while playing basketball.
PE	**Crescendo–decrescendo systolic ejection murmur to right of sternum and radiating to neck;** soft S2 with **paradoxical splitting** (due to aortic valve closure preceding pulmonary valve closure); weak and delayed carotid pulses.
Labs	ECG: left ventricular hypertrophy.
Imaging	CXR: calcifications on valve leaflets and enlarged cardiac shadow (due to large left ventricle). Echo: presence of bicuspid aortic valve.
Gross Pathology	Congenital bicuspid valve with calcification.
Micro Pathology	N/A
Treatment	Balloon valvuloplasty; surgical prosthetic replacement or changing of normal pulmonary valve to aortic site and insertion of pulmonary prosthesis (= ROSS PROCEDURE); antibiotic prophylaxis with penicillin prior to surgical or dental procedures.
Discussion	Causes include **congenital bicuspid aortic valve** (more common in males), **progressive degenerative calcification** of normal valves (more common in elderly males), and rheumatic heart disease (mitral valve is usually involved as well).

. . . .

AORTIC STENOSIS

ID/CC	A 59-year-old white male complains of **pain in the calf muscles** during exercise (= CLAUDICATION) along with coldness and numbness in both legs; his symptoms have been occurring for a year and are **relieved by rest.**
HPI	The patient has also been **impotent** and has been experiencing abdominal pain (due to mesenteric ischemia) about half an hour after eating (= POSTPRANDIAL PAIN). He **smokes** two packs of cigarettes a day.
PE	VS: **hypertension** (BP 150/100). PE: **diminished peripheral pulses** bilaterally; **loss of hair** over dorsum of feet and hands; decreased temperature in hands and feet; **carotid and femoral arterial bruits;** atrophy of calf muscles.
Labs	**Elevated LDL and decreased HDL;** elevated total serum cholesterol.
Imaging	Angio: multiple large **atheromatous plaques in aortoiliac distribution.** XR-Plain: irregular arterial vascular calcifications. US-Doppler: high-velocity poststenotic flow jet.
Gross Pathology	Early: fatty streak in endothelium; late: **fibrofatty plaque** formation with dystrophic calcification (atheroma) with narrowing of lumen of vessel wall.
Micro Pathology	Early: **foam cells** with intimal proliferation of smooth muscle cells; late: smooth muscle cells synthesize collagen and form **fibrous cap** with **necrotic lipid core** and fibrous plaque.
Treatment	Dietary modification; cholesterol-lowering drugs (e.g., lovastatin); angioplasty; coronary stenting; coronary artery bypass grafting (CABG).
Discussion	The main cause of coronary artery disease and the leading cause of mortality in the U.S.; also the cause of intestinal angina, peripheral vascular disease, cerebrovascular disease, and renovascular hypertension. **FIRST AID** p.243

ATHEROSCLEROSIS

ID/CC	A 47-year-old man complains of occasional **palpitations** and **shortness of breath.**
HPI	He also says that he occasionally experiences mild **dizziness** and chest discomfort.
PE	VS: **irregularly irregular** pulse. PE: variable-intensity S1 with occasional S3.
Labs	ECG: variable ventricular rate (80–200); can be > 200 with wide QRS if associated with accessory pathway; **no discernible P waves seen.** Normal CK-MB.
Imaging	CXR: normal.
Gross Pathology	N/A
Micro Pathology	N/A
Treatment	**Beta-blockers; calcium channel blockers; digitalis** (to decrease conduction at AV node in order to prevent ventricular arrhythmias); **electrical cardioversion** (if associated with ventricular tachycardia); patients should also be **anticoagulated** with warfarin to prevent embolic disease.
Discussion	The most common chronic arrhythmia, it is associated with a high risk of **embolic disease.** Causes include drugs, mitral valve disease, hypertensive and ischemic heart disease, dilated cardiomyopathy, alcoholism, **hyperthyroidism,** pericarditis, and cardiac surgery; it may also be idiopathic.

ATRIAL FIBRILLATION

ID/CC	A 65-year-old white male complains of **requiring three pillows in bed in order to breathe comfortably** (= ORTHOPNEA) and having to open the window to **gasp for air at night** (= PAROXYSMAL NOCTURNAL DYSPNEA).
HPI	He has also noted **increasing shortness of breath** while walking together with **swelling of his ankles and legs.** He had a **myocardial infarction** two years ago and has a history of **chronic hypertension.**
PE	VS: tachycardia; tachypnea; weak, thready pulse. PE: central cyanosis; **distention of neck veins** (due to elevated JVP); **third heart sound;** grade III/VI crescendo aortic systolic murmur; **crepitant rales** over both lower lobes; **lower lung fields dull to percussion** bilaterally; tender hepatomegaly; 4+ **pitting edema** in both lower extremities; cold extremities.
Labs	ABGs: hypoxemia; **low cardiac output** as measured by Fick equation and Swan–Ganz catheter (2.4 L/min); transudate in pleural fluid; increased BUN. ECG: left ventricular hypertrophy.
Imaging	CXR: enlarged cardiac silhouette; bilateral pleural effusions and diffuse increased lung markings (= KERLEY B LINES) suggesting pulmonary edema. Echo: **ejection fraction of 40%.**
Gross Pathology	Cardiomegaly due to both dilatation and hypertrophy; pulmonary edema with increase in weight and reddish-purple color; nutmeg liver (due to chronic passive congestion).
Micro Pathology	Hepatization of lungs with alveolar capillary congestion and alveolar macrophages with hemosiderin (= "HEART FAILURE CELLS"); centrilobular liver congestion.
Treatment	**Diuretics; low-sodium diet, digoxin;** ACE inhibitors; nitrates; antiarrhythmics.
Discussion	Heart failure due to a deficit in myocardial strength or an increase in workload. CHF is a common complication of ischemic and hypertensive heart disease in older populations. **FIRST AID** p.246

CONGESTIVE HEART FAILURE (CHF)

ID/CC	A 60-year-old white male who has been treated for **COPD** comes to the emergency room with severe **dyspnea at rest.**
HPI	Over the past few months, the patient has noted an **increased productive cough** and **exertional dyspnea.** He admits to being a **heavy smoker** and failed to quit smoking even after the appearance of **symptoms and the diagnosis of COPD.**
PE	Elevated JVP with large a and v waves; **loud P2;** cyanosis; clubbing of fingers; bilateral wheezing; expiratory rhonchi; prolonged expiration; use of accessory muscles of respiration; left parasternal heave; **ankle and sacral edema; tender hepatomegaly.**
Labs	ECG: **right axis deviation** and **peaked P waves** (= P PULMONALE). PFTs: COPD pattern.
Imaging	CXR: right ventricular and **pulmonary artery enlargement; hyperinflation.**
Gross Pathology	Right ventricular hypertrophy.
Micro Pathology	N/A
Treatment	Oxygen; salt and water restriction; treatment of COPD.
Discussion	**Right heart failure due to a pulmonary cause,** most commonly due to COPD. Other causes are pulmonary fibrosis, pneumoconioses, recurrent pulmonary embolism, primary pulmonary hypertension, obesity with sleep apnea, and kyphoscoliosis.

COR PULMONALE

ID/CC	A 29-year-old female who **recently gave birth** to a healthy infant develops **dyspnea** and **swelling of her feet** toward the end of the day.
HPI	She is nursing her six-week-old child.
PE	VS: BP mildly elevated. PE: JVP raised with prominent a and v waves; tender, mild hepatosplenomegaly; cardiac apex heaving and displaced outside midclavicular line; **pansystolic apical murmur** (due to **mitral insufficiency**) and systolic murmur increasing with inspiration heard in tricuspid area (due to tricuspid insufficiency); loud pulmonary component of S2; S3 and S4 gallop; fine inspiratory basal crepitant rales at both lung bases; pedal edema.
Labs	ECG: premature ventricular contractions.
Imaging	CXR: interstitial pulmonary edema (due to severe pulmonary venous hypertension); **global cardiomegaly.** Echo/Nuc: cardiomegaly with diminished ventricular contractility (**systolic dysfunction**). Stress Test: **decreased ejection fraction with stress** (ejection fraction normally increases with stress).
Gross Pathology	Global dilatation of all chambers.
Micro Pathology	**Extensive fibrosis without active inflammation** on endocardial biopsy.
Treatment	Cardiac failure treated with salt restriction, diuretics, vasodilators, and digoxin; chronic anticoagulation; nutritional supplementation; consider cardiac transplant if medical therapy fails.
Discussion	Usually develops in the **peripartum period** (± 3 months). Other etiologies include **alcoholism** (due to thiamine deficiency or direct toxicity), hypothyroidism, Friedreich's ataxia, previous **myocarditis** (usually due to coxsackie B), and drug toxicities, e.g., **adriamycin**, cyclophosphamide, **tricyclic antidepressants, lithium**, and cobalt. **FIRST AID** p.245

DILATED CARDIOMYOPATHY

ID/CC   A 21-year-old white male presents with anginal chest pain, **dyspnea on exertion,** and an episode of **syncope while playing basketball.**

HPI   The patient has no history of blue spells, squatting for relief, or rheumatic fever in childhood.

PE   VS: pulse bisferious (= DOUBLE PEAKED). PE: JVP normal; cardiac apex forceful with strong presystolic impulse (= DOUBLE APICAL IMPULSE); systolic thrill palpable over left sternal border; S4; **ejection systolic murmur** over left third intercostal space radiating to base and axilla; murmur **increased by exercise and during forced expiration against a closed glottis** (= VALSALVA MANEUVER) but **decreased by squatting.**

Labs   ECG: left axis deviation due to **left ventricular hypertrophy;** Q wave exaggerated in inferior and lateral precordial leads (due to septal hypertrophy).

Imaging   CXR-PA: often normal. Echo: **asymmetrical septal hypertrophy and systolic anterior motion of mitral valve;** doppler may show **mitral regurgitation.** Angio-Cardiac: marked **thickening of left ventricular septal wall;** small ventricular cavity with impaired ventricular filling (diastolic dysfunction) and narrow outflow tract (= "HOURGLASS" APPEARANCE).

Gross Pathology   **Enlarged heart** with increased weight and **asymmetrical septal hypertrophy.**

Micro Pathology   Myocyte disarray with increased norepinephrine content.

Treatment   Negative inotropic agents (e.g., **beta-blockers**) to decrease stiffness of left ventricle and prevent fatal arrhythmias; **avoidance of competitive sports;** amiodarone (may be useful in prevention of lethal cardiac arrhythmias); surgical myomectomy of interventricular septum in patients with outflow obstruction.

Discussion   Also known as **idiopathic hypertrophic subaortic stenosis (IHSS).** An **autosomal-dominant** pattern of disease is noted in 15% of cases; ventricular outflow tract obstruction by hypertrophy produces symptoms. The presenting symptom in **athletes** might be **sudden death** secondary to lethal cardiac arrhythmias. **FIRST AID** p.245

HYPERTROPHIC CARDIOMYOPATHY

ID/CC	A 42-year-old black male presents with **chest pain, headache, altered mental status, and confusion.**
HPI	He is known to have **labile essential hypertension.** He has no history of fever.
PE	VS: **severe diastolic hypertension** (BP 230/150). PE: **disoriented and confused; bilateral papilledema;** no focal neurologic deficits; remainder of exam normal.
Labs	CBC: microangiopathic hemolytic anemia. UA: **hematuria** and **proteinuria. Increased BUN and serum creatinine.** ECG: **left ventricular hypertrophy.**
Imaging	CT/US-Abdomen: bilateral **small and scarred kidneys.**
Gross Pathology	Kidney surface appears **"flea-bitten"** (due to underlying **necrotizing glomerulitis**).
Micro Pathology	Renal biopsy (not routinely indicated) shows **hyperplastic arteriolosclerosis** of vessels with fibrinoid necrosis (= "ONION SKINNING") and thrombi in vessel lumens.
Treatment	IV **sodium nitroprusside** or IV beta-blockers in conjunction with 24-hour cardiac monitoring in acute phase; subsequent management with oral antihypertensives and emphasis on strict patient compliance.
Discussion	**End-organ damage** caused by malignant hypertension includes hemorrhagic and lacunar strokes, encephalopathy, fundal hemorrhages, papilledema, myocardial ischemia/infarction, left ventricular hypertrophy, congestive heart failure, nephrosclerosis, azotemia, proteinuria, aortic dissection, and necrotizing vasculitis.

ID/CC	A 37-year-old white male complains of increasing **fatigue** and shortness of breath **during minimal physical exertion.**
HPI	He denies having had any chest pain or having any previous history of similar symptoms. A careful history reveals **rheumatic fever** at age seven.
PE	VS: jerky pulse (= RAPID UPSTROKE). PE: high-pitched **pansystolic murmur** at **apex with radiation to axilla;** S3.
Labs	ECG: left axis deviation; left atrial and left ventricular hypertrophy.
Imaging	CXR/Echo: enlargement of left atrium and ventricle. Doppler: confirmatory.
Gross Pathology	N/A
Micro Pathology	Aschoff bodies (lesions of fibrinoid necrosis surrounded by lymphocytes and histiocytes) if caused by rheumatic heart disease.
Treatment	Surgical repair or prosthetic replacement; antibiotic prophylaxis with penicillin prior to surgical or dental procedures.
Discussion	Common causes include **mitral valve prolapse,** ischemic papillary muscle dysfunction, and infective endocarditis; rheumatic heart disease is no longer the leading cause.

ID/CC	A 34-year-old white female in her 27th week of pregnancy is admitted to the hospital with **dyspnea** and **orthopnea.**
HPI	The patient denies any prior cardiovascular disease, but a careful history reveals that she suffered from **streptococcal pharyngitis** and **rheumatic heart disease** as a child.
PE	Malar flush; elevated JVP (due to venous congestion); left parasternal heave; loud S1; **opening snap;** rumbling, low-pitched **mid-diastolic murmur** at **apex** heard best in left lateral position.
Labs	ECG: **left atrial hypertrophy** and/or **atrial fibrillation.**
Imaging	CXR: double silhouette due to enlarged left atrium; Kerley B lines (due to interstitial edema). Echo: doppler confirmatory.
Gross Pathology	Thickened and scarred mitral valve.
Micro Pathology	N/A
Treatment	Treat atrial fibrillation; anticoagulation, commissurotomy, prosthetic valve replacement; antibiotic prophylaxis prior to surgical or dental procedures.
Discussion	The most common cause is rheumatic heart disease.

. . . .

MITRAL STENOSIS

ID/CC A 78-year-old white **male** is brought into the emergency room with **nausea, dyspnea,** and a **crushing substernal chest pain** that **radiates to** his **left arm and jaw**; the pain has lasted for about 30 minutes and is not relieved with rest.

HPI One sublingual tablet did not relieve his pain. His history reveals a **sedentary lifestyle, moderate hypercholesterolemia,** and **obesity.** The patient is also a **diabetic** and **smokes.**

PE VS: hypotension. PE: **diaphoresis.**

Labs ECG: **ST elevation** following **peaking of T waves;** subsequent development of Q waves and ultimately inverted T waves. **Elevated CK-MB; elevated troponin** T and I. CBC: leukocytosis.

Imaging Echo: **decreased wall motion** (= AKINESIS).

Gross Pathology 12 hours: no myocardial damage; 24 hours: pallor due to coagulation necrosis or reddish mottling; 3–5 days: demarcated yellow region with hyperemic border; 2–3 weeks: soft, gelatinous; 1–2 months: white scar and firm, thin wall.

Micro Pathology 12–18 hours: nuclear pyknosis, **coagulation necrosis,** and eosinophilia; 1–3 days: intense neutrophilic infiltrate, loss of nuclei and cross-striations; 1 week: disappearance of PMNs, onset of fibroblastic repair; 3 weeks: granulation tissue with progressive fibrosis.

Treatment **Thrombolysis** (with streptokinase or tPA), **percutaneous transluminal coronary angioplasty (PTCA), coronary artery bypass graft (CABG),** treat arrhythmias (lidocaine) and pain, oxygen, **aspirin,** antihypertensives, continuous cardiac monitoring.

Discussion The most common cause is atherosclerosis (coronary artery disease); less commonly caused by coronary vasospasm (Prinzmetal's angina). Sequelae include arrhythmias, congestive heart failure, pulmonary edema, shock, pulmonary embolism, papillary muscle rupture, ventricular aneurysm, ventricular wall rupture, tamponade, and autoimmune fibrinous pericarditis (= DRESSLER'S SYNDROME). **FIRST AID** p.244

· ·

MYOCARDIAL INFARCTION

ID/CC	A 64-year-old white female complains of **sudden-onset severe pain** in her left leg with **associated weakness** of the left foot. The pain intensifies when she moves her leg, and she cannot move her toes at all.
HPI	She is a **smoker** and has a history of **limited exercise tolerance** due to **pain in her lower extremities** (= INTERMITTENT CLAUDICATION).
PE	VS: normal. PE: lipid deposition in skin (= XANTHELASMAS); popliteal, dorsalis pedis, and posterior tibial **pulses lost** on left side; femoral pulses easily palpable; left leg **cold and mottled; anesthesia** over lower left leg.
Labs	CBC: leukocytosis.
Imaging	US-Doppler: obstruction of left femoral artery at origin. Angio: confirmatory; assess runoff and collaterals prior to surgery.
Gross Pathology	N/A
Micro Pathology	N/A
Treatment	Thrombolysis; consider embolectomy.
Discussion	Arterial embolism may have various causes, such as **atrial fibrillation, myocardial infarction, prosthetic heart valves,** or a dislodged mural thrombus from an **abdominal aortic aneurysm** or an atheromatous plaque. The earlier the intervention, the higher the likelihood that the limb may be salvaged. Clinically characterized by the **five P's: pain, pallor, paralysis, paresthesia, and pulselessness.**

ID/CC	A **30-year-old** white female is found to be **hypertensive** on routine physical exam.
HPI	She claims to have **no history of hypertension** and denies any changes in lifestyle or excessive stress.
PE	VS: **hypertension** (BP 175/105); PE: loud S2; funduscopic exam normal; **abdominal bruit** present.
Labs	**Elevated plasma renin.**
Imaging	Angio-Renal: confirmatory; unilateral left **renal artery stenosis in a "string of pearls" pattern.**
Gross Pathology	In fibromuscular dysplasia, the renal artery lumen is decreased due to hyperplastic fibrotic wall thickening.
Micro Pathology	Muscular hyperplasia with fibrosis and segmental stenosis.
Treatment	**ACE inhibitors** (contraindicated in bilateral renal artery stenosis). Balloon angioplasty; stenting; surgical correction.
Discussion	Secondary systemic hypertension caused by hypersecretion of renin from ischemic kidney. Most often caused by **fibromuscular dysplasia (young women)** or **atherosclerosis (older men)**; accounts for < 5% of all causes of hypertension.

· ·

RENOVASCULAR HYPERTENSION

ID/CC A 50-year-old male presents with complaints of **palpitations** and **chest pain.**

HPI The pain increases with physical activity and is relieved by rest. He has **multiple sexual partners.**

PE VS: high-volume, **collapsing pulse** (= WATER-HAMMER PULSE); **wide pulse pressure.** PE: pistol shots heard over brachial artery; to-and-fro murmur heard over femoral artery (= DUROZIEZ'S MURMUR); cardiomegaly; loud aortic component of S2; grade III **early diastolic murmur** heard radiating down right sternal edge (murmur of aortic incompetence); mid-diastolic murmur heard at apex (= AUSTIN FLINT MURMUR).

Labs ECG: **left ventricular hypertrophy** with strain pattern. **VDRL and FTA-ABS positive.**

Imaging CXR: **"tree bark" calcification** of ascending aorta and arch of aorta; **mediastinal widening and cardiomegaly.** Echo: **aortic incompetence;** left ventricular hypertrophy and dilatation.

Gross Pathology Gross cardiac hypertrophy (cor bovinum); **aortic** aneurysm involving the **arch** and the **ascending aorta** and extending into the aortic valve, rendering it incompetent.

Micro Pathology **Obliterative endarteritis** of vasa vasorum; degeneration and fibrosis of outer two-thirds of aortic media; compensatory irregular fibrous thickening of aortic intima.

Treatment Penicillin.

Discussion Aortitis occurs in the **tertiary stage of syphilis,** often arising many decades after the primary infection. Weakening of the aortic wall causes dilatation of the aortic root as well as aortic incompetence and aneurysms. Intimal fibrosis causes narrowing of the openings of the coronary arteries (ostial stenosis), resulting in myocardial ischemia.

· ·

SYPHILITIC AORTITIS

ID/CC	A 79-year-old white woman complains of a **throbbing, unilateral headache** that is most severe around her forehead and temples.
HPI	She has had recurrent bouts of **fever** over the past year and also complains of **malaise** and **muscle aches**. She reports some weight loss and occasional **vision problems** in her right eye. She also reports **pain in her mandible when she is eating** (= JAW CLAUDICATION).
PE	VS: fever. PE: **nodular enlargement of temporal artery with tenderness.**
Labs	CBC: normal WBC count; mild anemia. **Markedly elevated ESR,** usually > 100 mm/hour.
Imaging	N/A
Gross Pathology	Swollen, cordlike, segmentally nodular temporal artery.
Micro Pathology	**Granulomatous** inflammatory infiltrate of media and adventitia on **temporal artery biopsy;** fragmentation of elastica with multinucleated giant cells and fibrotic patches.
Treatment	Steroids should be started empirically before biopsy confirmation to **prevent blindness.**
Discussion	The most **common vasculitis** in the U.S., it frequently **coexists with polymyalgia rheumatica** and carries a risk of ipsilateral **blindness** due to thrombosis of the **ophthalmic artery.** Diagnosis and treatment are based on clinical grounds, since biopsy is positive in only 60% of cases. **FIRST AID** p.248

TEMPORAL ARTERITIS

ID/CC	A **35-year-old man** complains of severe, **cramping pains in his calves that prevent him from walking** (= INTERMITTENT CLAUDICATION).
HPI	The patient states that the pain comes mainly after playing basketball. More recently it has appeared, accompanied by numbness, following mild exertion and at rest (due to progression of disease). He admits to **smoking** up to three packs of cigarettes per day.
PE	Painful, cordlike indurations of veins (sequelae of migratory superficial thrombophlebitis); **pallor;** cyanosis; coldness; diminished peripheral artery pulsations; Raynaud's phenomenon; delayed return of hand color following release of temporarily occluded radial artery while exercising hand.
Labs	N/A
Imaging	Angio-Peripheral: **multiple occluded segments** of small and medium-sized arteries in lower leg.
Gross Pathology	Arterial segmental thrombosis; **no atherosclerosis;** secondary **gangrene** of leg if severe.
Micro Pathology	Segmental vasculitis with round cell infiltration in **all layers** of arterial wall; inflammation; thrombosis; microabscess formation.
Treatment	**Cessation of smoking** critical; sympathectomy; amputation.
Discussion	If smoking is not discontinued, multiple finger and toe amputations may be necessary. **FIRST AID** p.248

· ·

THROMBOANGIITIS OBLITERANS

ID/CC	A 60-year-old white male **farmer** presents with skin lesions on his **forehead, above his upper lip, and on the dorsum of his hands.**
HPI	He does not smoke, drink alcohol, or chew tobacco.
PE	Round or irregularly shaped lesions; tan plaques with adherent **scaly or rough surface** on forehead, skin over upper lip, forearms, and dorsum of hands; lesions range in size from several millimeters to 1 cm or more.
Labs	N/A
Imaging	N/A
Gross Pathology	N/A
Micro Pathology	Epidermis thickened with basal cell hyperplasia; atypical cells tend to invade most superficial portion of the dermis, which shows thickening and fibrosis (= ELASTOSIS).
Treatment	Liquid-nitrogen cryotherapy; topical treatment with fluorouracil; surgical excision; electrodesiccation.
Discussion	Also known as senile or **solar keratosis,** it is the most common **precancerous dermatosis** and may progress to **squamous cell carcinoma.** Signs that actinic keratosis has become malignant are elevation, ulceration or inflammation, and recent enlargement (> 1 cm). Immunosuppressed patients are at high risk of developing actinic keratosis with **prolonged sun exposure.** Look for multiple lesions and for newly developed lesions; **biopsy all suspicious lesions.**

ACTINIC KERATOSIS

ID/CC	A 68-year-old **red-haired white** male presents with a three-month history of a progressively **raised, bleeding, ulcerated lesion** over his upper lip that has not responded to various ointments.
HPI	He is a **farmer** and has always **worked outdoors**; he occasionally smokes but does not drink.
PE	Large, **ill-defined, telangiectatic and ulcerated nodule** (= "PEARLY PAPULE") with heaped-up borders located over right upper lip; no regional lymphadenopathy.
Labs	N/A
Imaging	N/A
Gross Pathology	Generally local but sometimes extensive destruction.
Micro Pathology	Biopsy shows basophilic cells with scant cytoplasm as well as palisading basal cells with atypia and increased mitotic index.
Treatment	Surgical excision with biopsy.
Discussion	Typically occurs in **light-skinned people. The most common skin cancer,** it is seen mainly on **sun-exposed areas** (e.g., face, nose) and is very slow-growing. **Metastatic disease is rare** (< 0.17%); **chronic, prolonged exposure to sun** is the most important risk factor. An increased incidence is seen in people with defective DNA repair mechanisms (e.g., xeroderma pigmentosum).

BASAL CELL CARCINOMA

ID/CC	A 23-year-old **HIV-positive** man presents with **nonpruritic reddish-brown lesions.**
HPI	He has had a continuous low-grade fever, significant weight loss over the past six months, and painless lumps in the cervical, axillary, and inguinal areas.
PE	VS: fever. PE: emaciation; pallor; generalized lymphadenopathy; no hepatosplenomegaly or sternal tenderness; **reddish-purple plaques and nodules** over trunk and lower extremities; similar lesions noted in oral mucosa.
Labs	ELISA/Western blot positive for HIV. CBC/PBS: **lymphocytopenia with depressed CD4+ cell count** (< 100).
Imaging	N/A
Gross Pathology	Reddish-purple plaques and firm nodules with no suppuration.
Micro Pathology	Skin biopsy shows malignant spindle cells with slitlike spaces containing RBCs, hemosiderin, and inflammatory cells.
Treatment	Chemotherapy with etoposide or doxorubicin, bleomycin, and vinblastine. If iatrogenic, stop immunosuppressive medication.
Discussion	The **most common cancer associated with AIDS.** The non-AIDS type affects Ashkenazi Jews and Africans, but the disease is not as aggressive. **Human herpesvirus 8** is associated with all types.

ID/CC	A 50-year-old **white** male presents with an itchy, **rapidly enlarging, pigmented lesion** on the sole of his left foot.
HPI	He states that the spot has **recently changed color** dramatically; once lightly pigmented, it is now a deep purple hue.
PE	**Irregular, asymmetric, deeply pigmented lesion with various shades** of red and blue; diameter **> 6 mm**; left-sided nontender **inguinal lymphadenopathy.**
Labs	N/A
Imaging	N/A
Gross Pathology	**Slightly raised;** deeply pigmented with uneven hues and irregular border.
Micro Pathology	Excisional biopsy shows tumor-free borders along with large, atypical, variably pigmented cells with irregular nuclei and eosinophilic nucleoli in epidermis and papillary dermis; dermal invasion noted in some places; metastases shown on lymph node biopsy.
Treatment	Excision with wide margin, regional lymph node dissection, chemotherapy, immunotherapy.
Discussion	Of all skin cancers, melanoma is responsible for the largest number of deaths. An increased incidence is seen in **fair-skinned** people and in those with **dysplastic nevi** and **excessive sun exposure.** The **chance of metastasis increases with depth of invasion** (measured using Clark levels I–V). **FIRST AID** p.224

ID/CC   A 60-year-old male presents with multiple lumps and a **chronic,** pruritic, erythematous **rash** that has spread and now **involves almost his entire body.**

HPI   He has seen many doctors, but the rash **has not responded to** a variety of medications, including **topical and systemic steroids.**

PE   Erythematous, circinate rash in **plaques** with **exfoliation** (= SCALING); some **nodules** seen on face, trunk, lower abdomen, and buttocks; no regional lymphadenopathy or hepatosplenomegaly.

Labs   CBC/PBS: lymphocytosis.

Imaging   CXR: no mediastinal lymphadenopathy.

Gross Pathology   Reddish-brown, **kidney-shaped plaques** (vs. Hodgkin's lymphoma); hence name **"red man's disease"**; exfoliation, nodule formation, and sometimes ulceration.

Micro Pathology   Atypical, **PAS-positive, large lymphocytes with characteristic multiconvoluted, "cerebriform" nuclei** (= SÉZARY-LUTZNER CELLS); dermal infiltration with exocytosis of atypical mononuclear cells within epidermis found singly or within punched-out **epidermal microabscesses** (= PAUTRIER'S ABSCESSES).

Treatment   PUVA; total skin electron-beam therapy; prednisone and chlorambucil or low-dose methotrexate.

Discussion   Malignant cutaneous helper T-cell lymphoma; disseminated disease with exfoliative dermatitis and generalized lymphadenopathy is termed **Sézary syndrome.**

· ·

MYCOSIS FUNGOIDES

ID/CC	A 6-year-old boy is brought in for a pediatric consultation due to a hoarse voice, **growth retardation,** and developmental delay.
HPI	The boy's mother describes a **prolonged gestation** and a birth weight of 4.5 kg. The boy has had problems at school owing to a short attention span, sleeping in class, and **mental sluggishness.**
PE	Dry, **yellowish skin;** wide-based ataxic gait; **large tongue** (= MACROGLOSSIA); muscular atrophy; **short stature** for age; broad nose; **umbilical hernia;** puffy eyes (due to myxedema) and wide epicanthal distance; slow relaxation of tendon reflexes; thin, brittle hair; **protuberant abdomen;** weak, hoarse voice.
Labs	Elevated TSH; low T3 and T4.
Imaging	XR-Plain: absence of some ossification centers; coxa vara (= DECREASED FEMORAL ANGLE); delayed epiphyseal development.
Gross Pathology	Enlarged thyroid gland; **myxedema;** failure of sexual organs to develop properly.
Micro Pathology	N/A
Treatment	Levothyroxine replacement.
Discussion	**Congenital hypothyroidism** in an infant or child leads to **irreversible mental retardation;** it is caused by lack of iodine, thyroid developmental defects, radioactive iodine exposure during pregnancy, autoimmune disorders, and drugs. Protean manifestations include neuromuscular impairment, short stature (dwarfism), cardiovascular symptoms, and **sexual retardation;** can be **mistaken for Down's syndrome** with grave consequences. All states in the U.S. currently require neonatal screening for hypothyroidism, galactosemia, and phenylketonuria. **FIRST AID** p.239

CRETINISM

ID/CC	An obese **44-year-old female** complains of **irritability** and excessive weight gain (40 kg) over the past three years and requests medical weight-loss therapy.
HPI	On careful questioning, she also reports **easy bruising, oligomenorrhea, weakness, and increased hair growth** in various areas of her body.
PE	VS: hypertension (BP 180/110). PE: facial acne; **truncal obesity** with thin extremities; **buffalo hump** and plethoric **moon facies; hirsutism;** wide, purple abdominal and lower leg **striae.**
Labs	UA: 3+ glucosuria. **Elevated fasting blood sugar; elevated plasma cortisol;** high ACTH. Lytes: **hypokalemia.** CBC: leukopenia. **Dexamethasone suppression test** suppressed hypercortisolism.
Imaging	XR-Plain: **generalized osteoporosis.**
Gross Pathology	Pituitary adenoma; bilateral **adrenocortical hyperplasia.**
Micro Pathology	Pituitary: benign basophilic adenoma with Crook's hyalinization.
Treatment	Surgical removal of pituitary adenoma (transsphenoidal adenectomy) or pituitary irradiation along with adjunct medical therapy.
Discussion	Cushing's syndrome comprises the manifestations of hypercortisolism regardless of its cause; Cushing's disease is due to increased ACTH production by the pituitary.

ID/CC	An **8-year-old** black male is brought to his pediatrician because of a 4-kg **weight loss** over a period of three months.
HPI	His mother says that he has also been complaining of **excessive thirst, hunger, and urination** (= POLYDIPSIA, POLYPHAGIA, POLYURIA). The patient also reports **waking up several times during the night to urinate** (= NOCTURIA).
PE	**Thinly built** male child with an otherwise normal physical exam.
Labs	Elevated **fasting blood sugar** (180 mg/dL); elevated postprandial blood sugar (270 mg/dL). UA: **glycosuria. Islet cell antibodies** and **anti-insulin antibodies in serum;** elevated glycosylated hemoglobin (**hemoglobin A$_{1C}$**).
Imaging	N/A
Gross Pathology	N/A
Micro Pathology	Decreased number of pancreatic beta islets with hyalinization, fibrosis, and lymphocytic infiltration.
Treatment	Insulin (type I diabetics do not have circulating insulin and require exogenous insulin to **prevent diabetic ketoacidosis**), sugar-restricted diet.
Discussion	**Insulin-dependent diabetes mellitus** (IDDM), or **type I,** is caused by **autoimmune** destruction of beta cells. It may be triggered by coxsackievirus B4, mumps, or other viruses in individuals with a genetic predisposition, and it is linked to **chromosome 6 - HLA-DR3 or -DR4.** Close-to-normal values of **glycosylated hemoglobin** reflect good long-term control of blood sugar levels. **FIRST AID** p.240

DIABETES MELLITUS TYPE I

ID/CC	An **obese 55-year-old** white male complains of increasing **thirst** and **excessive appetite.**
HPI	He also complains of **increased urinary volume,** weight loss, and weakness over the past several months together with burning and **tingling sensations** in a **stocking-glove distribution** (due to peripheral neuropathy). His father was diabetic with a history of leg amputation and kidney failure.
PE	VS: hypertension (BP 150/95). PE: **"dot-blot" hemorrhages, exudates, and microaneurysms** on funduscopic exam; muscle atrophy in hips and thighs; diminished dorsalis pedis and tibialis pulses bilaterally.
Labs	Elevated (= HEMOGLOBIN A_{1c}) glycosylated hemoglobin. UA: **glucosuria.** Elevated fasting serum glucose.
Imaging	N/A
Gross Pathology	N/A
Micro Pathology	Amyloidosis; hyaline atherosclerosis; nodular hyaline masses (= KIMMELSTIEL–WILSON NODULES) in glomerulus.
Treatment	Diet and exercise; oral hypoglycemic agents; insulin as needed.
Discussion	Also known as **non-insulin-dependent diabetes mellitus (NIDDM),** it is a metabolic disease involving carbohydrates and lipids caused by peripheral **resistance to insulin.** Although patients with type II diabetes mellitus are not prone to developing diabetic ketoacidosis, they can develop **nonketotic hyperosmolar coma** if their blood glucose is drastically elevated. Sequelae of type I and type II diabetes mellitus include peripheral vascular disease, coronary artery disease, stroke, diabetic nephropathy, diabetic neuropathy, nonhealing skin ulcers, and delayed wound healing with increased risk of infection. **FIRST AID** p.240

DIABETES MELLITUS TYPE II

ID/CC	A 45-year-old woman presents with a **swelling in the anterior portion of her neck.**
HPI	She also complains of **slowed speech, easy fatigability,** and **cold intolerance.** She is known to have **rheumatoid arthritis,** for which she is taking NSAIDs.
PE	**Puffy face; dry skin; coarse hair; swelling of thyroid gland** in anterior portion of neck; swelling is mobile with deglutition but not with protrusion of tongue; thyroid has rubbery consistency; right lobe more enlarged than left; swan neck deformity of left ring finger; ulnar deviation of fingers of both hands.
Labs	**T3, T4 low;** TSH high; **anti-thyroglobulin antibodies** and thyroid **antimicrosomal antibodies** detected by ELISA.
Imaging	Nuc: decreased radioactive iodine uptake (RAIU).
Gross Pathology	Diffuse, moderate enlargement of thyroid gland; cut surface is light gray and appears similar to a lymph node.
Micro Pathology	Biopsy shows massive infiltration by lymphocytes and plasma cells; normal follicles not present; scant colloid; Hürthle cell degeneration seen.
Treatment	Replacement therapy with **levothyroxine (T4).**
Discussion	Often associated with other autoimmune diseases, including systemic lupus erythematosus, pernicious anemia, Sjögren's syndrome, and chronic hepatitis; has a genetic association with HLA-DR5 (goitrous form) and HLA-DR3 (atrophic form). Thyrotoxicosis may be seen early in the course of this **autoimmune disease** (hashitoxicosis).

. . . .

HASHIMOTO'S THYROIDITIS

ID/CC	A 24-year-old white female comes to her family doctor because of **weight loss** despite having a **good appetite**; she also complains of increasing **anxiety**.
HPI	She admits to having frequent bouts of **diarrhea**, reduced sleep capacity, **heat intolerance**, sweaty palms, **palpitations**, **tremors**, and **menstrual irregularity**.
PE	VS: **tachycardia**. PE: tremors of outstretched hand; **warm, moist skin; right lobe of thyroid palpably enlarged; left lobe not palpable;** no evidence of retrosternal goiter; no cervical lymphadenopathy.
Labs	Increased T4 (= TOTAL PLASMA THYROXINE); increased resin triiodothyronine uptake (RT$_3$U); **decreased plasma TSH**.
Imaging	XR-Soft Tissue: no calcification in area of thyroid. CXR: no mediastinal mass. Nuc: **hyperfunctioning hot** (increased uptake) thyroid **nodule** with **decreased uptake in surrounding tissue and other lobe** (due to atrophy of remainder of gland secondary to feedback inhibition of TSH).
Gross Pathology	Smooth, rounded, well-circumscribed single mass in left lobe of thyroid gland; no areas of hemorrhage or necrosis; remainder of gland atrophic.
Micro Pathology	No signs of atypia; follicular stroma with abundant, normal-appearing colloid.
Treatment	Treatment of thyrotoxicosis with **propranolol** and antithyroid medications (e.g., propylthiouracil and methimazole); ablation of adenoma by either radioactive iodine or surgery.
Discussion	Plummer's nodule is a variant of toxic nodular goiter in which hyperthyroidism is caused by overproduction of thyroid hormone by a single thyroid adenoma known as **toxic adenoma.** **FIRST AID** p.241

HYPERTHYROIDISM (SOLITARY NODULE)

ID/CC	A 29-year-old white female is brought into the emergency room following a **seizure** on her way to work.
HPI	The patient underwent **thyroid surgery** for papillary cancer two years ago. She has been suffering from lethargy, **circumoral and foot numbness**, hand **fasciculations**, and **cramping** pain in the calves. Her family describes her as having been **irritable** and depressed over the past few months.
PE	Facial muscle contraction on tapping of facial nerve (= CHVOSTEK'S SIGN); **carpopedal spasm following application of blood pressure cuff** (= TROUSSEAU'S SIGN); brittle nails with fungal infection; coarse, scaly skin; cataracts.
Labs	Low calcium; elevated inorganic phosphorus; low magnesium; low PTH; normal alkaline phosphatase; low urine phosphorus and calcium.
Imaging	CT-Head: calcifications of the basal ganglia.
Gross Pathology	N/A
Micro Pathology	N/A
Treatment	Calcium; vitamin D; treat hypomagnesemia.
Discussion	Most commonly caused by **thyroidectomy** with removal of the parathyroid glands; symptoms are due to **hypocalcemia.**

· ·

HYPOPARATHYROIDISM

ID/CC	A 53-year-old female complains of **increasing fatigue, insomnia, and depression.**
HPI	For the past six months she has had episodes in which her **face and neck have become hot and red** (= HOT FLASHES). She has been **amenorrheic for the past seven months;** prior to this, her menstrual history was normal.
PE	**Thinning of the skin; hirsutism; atrophic vaginal mucosa** with decreased secretions.
Labs	Increased 24-hour urinary gonadotropins (LH and FSH).
Imaging	XR-Plain: **osteoporosis** of thoracolumbar spine.
Gross Pathology	N/A
Micro Pathology	N/A
Treatment	**Estrogen replacement therapy** beneficial.
Discussion	The estrogen-deficiency state produced by menopause has short-range (hot flashes), medium-range (vaginal atrophy), and long-range (osteoporosis) consequences that can be relieved or prevented by estrogen replacement. Common side effects in patients taking hormone replacement therapy include irregular bleeding, weight gain, fluid retention, and endometrial hyperplasia. Nevertheless, postmenopausal bleeding should be worked up with an endometrial biopsy to rule out endometrial cancer.

· ·

MENOPAUSE

ID/CC	A 42-year-old female is discovered to have **hypertension** on a routine physical exam.
HPI	She had been suffering from headaches, **weakness,** and leg cramps. A careful history discloses that she has also had **increased urinary volume.**
PE	VS: hypertension (BP 165/110). PE: diminished deep tendon reflexes.
Labs	Lytes: **hypokalemic alkalosis; high serum sodium** (154); **low serum potassium** (2.4). ECG: flattened T waves, long Q-T, U waves. **Increased urinary aldosterone; low plasma renin.**
Imaging	CT: small left adrenocortical adenoma. Angio-Abdomen: unequal aldosterone levels on adrenal vein sampling.
Gross Pathology	A 1.7-cm, nodular, nonencapsulated adenoma on left adrenal cortex.
Micro Pathology	Clear cells filled with foamy cytoplasm containing lipid vesicles intermixed with compact cells without cytoplasmic lipid.
Treatment	Adenoma: laparoscopic adrenalectomy. Hyperplasia: spironolactone; antihypertensive drugs.
Discussion	The most common cause of primary aldosteronism is a unilateral **adrenal cortex adenoma** (= CONN'S SYNDROME); less commonly caused by **adrenocortical hyperplasia.** Excessive aldosterone secretion results in hypertension, hypernatremia, and hypokalemia.

PRIMARY HYPERALDOSTERONISM

ID/CC	A 56-year-old white **female** complains of **severe, colicky left flank pain** radiating to the groin and inner thigh and associated with **nausea, vomiting,** and bloody urine.
HPI	She has a history of **burning epigastric pain** that is relieved by food. Her history also reveals anorexia, **confusion, irritability, constipation,** easy fatigability, **excessive thirst, and polyuria.**
PE	**Calcium deposits in cornea** (= BAND KERATOPATHY); left flank tenderness; thick fingernails; decreased muscle tone.
Labs	UA: hematuria; **elevated urine calcium and phosphorus.** ECG: short Q-T. Lytes: **elevated serum calcium and alkaline phosphatase; low serum phosphorus; elevated PTH.**
Imaging	KUB: **stone** in left renal pelvis. XR-Plain: **subperiosteal resorption** of bone in fingers and teeth; **chondrocalcinosis; multiple cystic bone lesions** (= OSTEITIS FIBROSA CYSTICA).
Gross Pathology	Adenoma: usually involvement of one gland only; hyperplasia: all four glands enlarged; **metastatic calcification** may involve many sites, including lungs.
Micro Pathology	Adenoma: involvement of chief cells compressing surrounding gland, producing atrophy; hyperplasia: involvement of chief or clear cells (wasserhelle type); lack of normal fat tissue.
Treatment	Surgical exploration and biopsy; parathyroidectomy; rule out malignancy.
Discussion	Most commonly caused by **adenomas; hyperplasia** and **malignancy** are less common causes. Usually asymptomatic and discovered on routine lab check-up. Symptoms result from hypercalcemia and include renal stones, polyuria, bone pain, constipation, nausea, vomiting, lethargy, peptic ulcers, mental status changes, and pancreatitis.

PRIMARY HYPERPARATHYROIDISM

ID/CC	A 33-year-old white female presents with **menstrual cycle irregularity** with long periods of **amenorrhea** and **milky nipple discharge** (= GALACTORRHEA).
HPI	Further questioning discloses that she has also **been unable to conceive.**
PE	VS: normotension. PE: no gynecological masses palpable; pelvic exam normal.
Labs	**Hyperprolactinemia; reduced LH and estradiol.**
Imaging	MR: enhancing pituitary microadenoma (< 10 mm); deviation of pituitary stalk.
Gross Pathology	N/A
Micro Pathology	N/A
Treatment	Bromocriptine (dopamine analog); consider transsphenoidal surgery.
Discussion	The most common type of pituitary adenoma. GnRH is suppressed by excessive prolactin secretion by the tumor, and thus LH and estradiol are reduced. In **males,** it presents with **headache, impotence,** and **visual disturbance.**

· · · · · · · · · · · · · · · · · ·

PROLACTINOMA

ID/CC	A 30-year-old **woman** presents with fatigue, **significant weight loss,** and **amenorrhea** of two years' duration.
HPI	She had a baby two years ago and suffered **significant postpartum bleeding**. She bottle-fed her baby because she was **unable to lactate** after delivery.
PE	VS: **hypotension** (BP 85/60). PE: skin tenting; fine wrinkling around eyes and mouth; loss of axillary and pubic hair.
Labs	**Decreased levels of trophic hormones (FSH, LH, ACTH, TSH);** decreased levels of target gland hormones (T3, T4, cortisol, estrogens).
Imaging	MR-Pituitary (usually before and after injection of gadolinium DTPA): abnormal signal in pituitary gland.
Gross Pathology	Soft, pale, and hemorrhagic pituitary gland in early stages; shrunken, fibrous, and firm in later stages.
Micro Pathology	N/A
Treatment	Hormone replacement: cortisol; levothyroxine (T4); estrogen-progesterone replacement.
Discussion	Sheehan's syndrome is most commonly caused by **postpartum infarction of the pituitary.** During delivery, loss of blood or hypovolemia decreases flow to the pituitary and leads to ischemia. Loss of trophic hormones leads to atrophy of target organs. This syndrome may also occur in males and in nonpregnant females (trauma, sickle cell anemia, disseminated intravascular coagulation, vascular accidents).

. . . .

SHEEHAN'S SYNDROME

ID/CC	A 50-year-old **female** presents with a **nodule in the front of her neck** that she first noticed one month ago.
HPI	She notes that the nodule has grown, but she does not complain of any symptoms suggestive of a hyperthyroid or hypothyroid state. She consumes iodized salt. She works as an **x-ray technician** (radiation exposure).
PE	**Firm, nontender nodule** in anterior portion of neck, mobile with deglutition; anterior cervical lymphadenopathy; no tremors, sweating, pretibial/pedal myxedema, or exophthalmos.
Labs	**Normal thyroid function tests;** normal thyroid hormone levels.
Imaging	XR-Neck: stippled calcification. Nuc: **cold nodule.** US: **solid nodule.**
Gross Pathology	Nodule can range in size from microscopic to several centimeters with invasive margins; may be sclerotic or partly cystic.
Micro Pathology	FNA: **psammoma bodies;** lymphocytes; large pink follicular cells with large, pale nuclei and numerous nucleoli.
Treatment	Ipsilateral lobectomy and exploration of regional lymph nodes; follow-up levels of serum thyroglobulin; levothyroxine suppression.
Discussion	**Ionizing radiation** is a predisposing factor for the development of **papillary carcinoma** of the thyroid. Papillary carcinoma spreads via the lymphatics and may present with only cervical lymphadenopathy and an occult primary. Of all histologic variants of thyroid cancer (papillary, follicular, mixed, medullary), papillary carcinoma carries the best prognosis. Medullary carcinoma of the thyroid is associated with multiple endocrine neoplasia (MEN) types IIa and IIb.

. . . .

THYROID CARCINOMA

ID/CC	A 33-year-old female complains of **increasing substernal pain and difficulty swallowing** liquids and solids (= DYSPHAGIA) over the past several months.
HPI	She has lost 20 pounds in the past three months and has occasionally experienced acute substernal pain and **regurgitation of food** into her mouth when lying down.
PE	Unremarkable.
Labs	Esophageal manometry reveals aperistaltic esophagus; **increased lower esophageal sphincter pressure;** negative antinuclear antibodies (ANAs) (vs. scleroderma).
Imaging	UGI: "rat-tailed" lower esophageal segment; dilatation; uncoordinated peristalsis. EGD: gaping cavity filled with dirty fluid. CXR: air–fluid level in enlarged esophagus.
Gross Pathology	Massive dilatation of esophagus (due to defect in esophageal peristalsis and/or **impaired relaxation of lower esophageal sphincter** during swallowing).
Micro Pathology	Loss of number of ganglion cells in myenteric plexus (similar to Hirschsprung's disease of the colon).
Treatment	Heller's esophagocardiomyotomy.
Discussion	Achalasia is a motility disorder of the esophagus due to **loss of ganglion cells in Auerbach's plexus.** Complications include candidal esophagitis, diverticula, and/or aspiration pneumonia. **FIRST AID** p.228

. . . .

ACHALASIA

ID/CC	A 42-year-old white female, the **mother of five**, develops **acute intermittent pain in the right upper quadrant** and right scapula **after eating a fatty meal.**
HPI	She is of **Native American ancestry** and is 30 pounds **overweight.** She also complains of **nausea** and has **vomited** three times. She has had several prior episodes of similar pain following meals.
PE	VS: fever. PE: **obese;** tenderness in right upper abdominal quadrant with **inspiratory arrest on palpation** (= MURPHY'S SIGN); hypoactive bowel sounds.
Labs	Hypercholesterolemia. CBC: **leukocytosis with mild neutrophilia.** Elevated direct bilirubin; **elevated alkaline phosphatase.**
Imaging	US: distended gallbladder with **wall thickening** containing **multiple echogenic shadows** (stones). Nuc-HIDA: failure to visualize gallbladder indicates cystic duct obstruction by stone.
Gross Pathology	Gallbladder inflammation ranging from wall edema to acute gangrene with necrosis, pus formation, and perforation with peritonitis. Most stones composed of **cholesterol;** less common are **pigmented stones** made principally of bilirubin.
Micro Pathology	Gallbladder mucosa contains lipid-laden foamy macrophages.
Treatment	Conservative treatment includes nasogastric aspiration, IV fluids, analgesics, and antibiotics; cholecystectomy (usually laparoscopic) definitive treatment.
Discussion	Differential diagnosis includes appendicitis, pancreatitis, perforated peptic ulcer, pyelonephritis, myocardial infarction, and right lower lobe pneumonia. Clinical risk factors include the **four F's: fat, female, forty, and fertile.**

. . . .

ACUTE CHOLECYSTITIS

ID/CC	A 37-year-old male **alcoholic** suddenly develops **nausea and vomiting** with diffuse **epigastric pain** and **"coffee-ground" vomitus** (blood reacts with gastric hydrochloric acid).
HPI	He **drank heavily** and **did not eat** anything for two days as part of a New Year's celebration. He also smokes two packs of cigarettes a day. He has been taking **aspirin** to relieve his headache.
PE	VS: **tachycardia; hypotension.** PE: pallor; skin cold and clammy; tenderness in midepigastrium; no peritoneal irritation; no lymphadenopathy; placement of nasogastric tube returned sanguinous fluid.
Labs	CBC/PBS: microcytic, hypochromic **anemia. Positive stool guaiac test** (occult blood in feces).
Imaging	UGI: **erosions and fold thickening** of gastric antrum. EGD: **petechial hemorrhages and small erosions** of gastric mucosa.
Gross Pathology	N/A
Micro Pathology	Focal necrosis of mucosa with acute inflammation (PMNs) and superficial ulceration on stomach biopsy.
Treatment	Stop alcohol consumption; bland diet; adequate hydration; liquid antacids; H₂ antagonists (e.g., cimetidine); proton pump inhibitors (e.g., omeprazole); blood transfusion and vasopressin infusion may be necessary to control and stabilize patient with massive GI bleeding.
Discussion	Predisposing factors include consumption of **irritating or corrosive substances, steroids, alcohol, aspirin, and other NSAIDs** as well as psychological **stress.**

ACUTE HEMORRHAGIC GASTRITIS

ID/CC	A 40-year-old male presents with **cramping abdominal pain** and **vomiting** of three hours' duration.
HPI	He also complains of an **inability to pass stool or flatus** (= OBSTIPATION) for the past three days. Two years ago, he underwent an emergency appendectomy for a ruptured appendix.
PE	Dehydration; **abdominal distention;** generalized mild tenderness over abdomen without rebound or guarding; bowel sounds heard as **high-pitched tinkles during pain paroxysms.**
Labs	CBC/PBS: leukocytosis with hemoconcentration. Serum amylase levels normal.
Imaging	XR-Abdomen: ladder-like pattern of multiple **dilated loops of small bowel** and **multiple air–fluid levels; colon and rectum gasless** (air in colon or rectum would indicate an intestinal ileus); no free air under diaphragm.
Gross Pathology	N/A
Micro Pathology	N/A
Treatment	IV fluid replacement; nasogastric suction/decompression; broad-spectrum antibiotics; surgery.
Discussion	The most common causes of small bowel obstruction are intestinal **adhesions secondary to prior abdominal surgery, neoplasms,** and incarcerated **hernia;** the most common causes of large bowel obstruction are carcinoma, volvulus, and adhesions. Complications include strangulation and necrosis of the bowel wall leading to perforation, peritonitis, and even sepsis.

. . . .

ACUTE INTESTINAL OBSTRUCTION

ID/CC A 34-year-old **alcoholic** male complains of sudden-onset **midepigastric pain radiating to the lower thoracic spine.**

HPI He also complains of associated **anorexia, nausea,** and **vomiting.**

PE VS: **hypotension; tachycardia.** PE: pale, sweaty; in severe distress; **periumbilical ecchymoses** (= CULLEN'S SIGN); **left flank ecchymosis** (= GREY TURNER'S SIGN); marked **epigastric tenderness** and diffuse **rebound tenderness** but minimal rigidity; abdomen distended with markedly decreased bowel sounds.

Labs **Markedly elevated serum amylase** and **lipase; elevated glucose;** elevated SGOT and LDH; **hypocalcemia.** ABGs: hypoxia.

Imaging CXR/KUB: no free air under diaphragm; abrupt termination of gaseous transverse colon at splenic flexure (= COLON CUTOFF SIGN); distended loop of bowel in proximal jejunum (= SENTINEL LOOP). CT-Abdomen: enlargement and **inhomogeneity** of pancreas; **streaky peripancreatic inflammation.**

Gross Pathology Autopsy: pancreas reveals pasty white foci of fat necrosis, hemorrhage, and cystic cavitation.

Micro Pathology Edema of connective tissue, polymorphonuclear infiltration, hemorrhage and necrosis of pancreatic acini; fat necrosis appears as pale blue amorphous foci where adipocyte membranes are dissolved.

Treatment Supportive management.

Discussion **Gallstones** and **alcohol abuse** are etiologic factors in 90% of patients with acute pancreatitis. Gallstones are thought to cause pancreatitis by **transient obstruction at the ampulla of Vater,** which leads to pancreatic ductal hypertension.

. . . .

ACUTE PANCREATITIS

ID/CC	A 61-year-old white male in apparent good health has a routine annual physical exam that reveals a small rectal mass.
HPI	He has no major complaints except for intermittent, mild diarrhea.
PE	**Mobile, nonpainful rectal mass** on digital rectal exam with no evidence of bleeding; examination otherwise unremarkable.
Labs	CBC: **anemia** (Hb 9.2/Hct 26.9). **Hemoccult-positive stool.**
Imaging	Sigmoidoscopy/BE: multiple **pedunculated masses** in sigmoid and transverse colon.
Gross Pathology	Discrete mass lesions from colonic epithelium protruding into intestinal lumen; vast majority measure < 2 cm, although may reach up to 5 cm; may have stalk (= PEDUNCULATED) or have a broad base (= SESSILE); may be **tubular, villous,** or **tubulovillous.**
Micro Pathology	Frequent mitosis, cellular atypia, and loss of normal polarity in intestinal epithelium of glands.
Treatment	Colonoscopic biopsy and removal; repeat colonoscopy or barium enema for periodic surveillance.
Discussion	The most common variety is adenomatous; the **risk of malignant transformation increases with size** and is **greatest in villous adenomas.** May be familial (familial adenomatous polyposis).

. . . .

ADENOMATOUS POLYPOSIS COLI

ID/CC	A 32-year-old homeless white male is brought to the emergency room by an ambulance following **convulsions** that took place on the street.
HPI	The patient is disheveled and unshaven in his appearance. A history cannot be obtained because he is alone and unable to respond to questions.
PE	Dehydration; **jaundice; alcohol on breath;** 2-cm laceration on occipital area with no bleeding; semicomatose state with response to pain only; pupils equal; **fine tremor** in extremities; palmar erythema; **hepatomegaly.**
Labs	CBC/PBS: **macrocytic, hypochromic anemia. Elevated** direct and indirect **bilirubin; elevated AST and ALT;** AST/ALT ratio of 2:1; **elevated alkaline phosphatase; elevated PT; low** serum **albumin;** hypoglycemia.
Imaging	N/A
Gross Pathology	**Fatty liver;** micronodular **cirrhosis;** marked **gastritis;** bronchial aspiration.
Micro Pathology	Hepatocytes distended with fat; hepatocellular necrosis; **Mallory bodies** (hyaline); cytoplasmic vacuolization of stem cells in bone marrow; myofibrillar necrosis; diffuse axonal degeneration.
Treatment	Vitamins (thiamine and folate); glucose; rehydration; treat acute withdrawal and delirium tremens (DTs) with benzodiazepines.
Discussion	Alcoholic **DTs** usually occur 2–5 days after cessation of drinking and are characterized by seizures, delusions, agitation, disorientation, visual and tactile hallucinations, and autonomic instability. DT prophylaxis consists of benzodiazepines and restraints to prevent damage to patient and to others. DTs have a mortality rate of 15% if untreated. **FIRST AID** p.249

· ·

ALCOHOLISM

ID/CC	A 17-year-old male student presents with anorexia and cramplike **periumbilical pain followed by nausea** and two episodes of **vomiting.**
HPI	Four hours after presentation, the **pain shifted to the right lower quadrant** and he developed a **low-grade fever.**
PE	VS: mild tachycardia; low-grade fever. PE: **right lower quadrant tenderness with guarding and rebound;** pain in right lower quadrant when pressure applied to left lower quadrant (= ROVSING'S SIGN); **pain localized to junction of outer and middle third of the line from anterior superior iliac spine to umbilicus** (= MCBURNEY'S POINT); right lower quadrant pain elicited by passive hip extension (= PSOAS SIGN) and by passive internal rotation of hip (= OBTURATOR SIGN).
Labs	CBC: **elevated WBC count; predominance of neutrophils.** Normal serum amylase. UA: normal.
Imaging	KUB: right psoas shadow blurred; generalized ileus with air–fluid levels; increased soft tissue density in right lower quadrant; small radiopaque **fecalith** in right lower quadrant. US: **noncompressible tubular structure** in right lower quadrant.
Gross Pathology	Early lesion: hyperemic appendix with fibrinous exudate; late lesion: purulent exudate with necrosis and perforation; fecalith occasionally present.
Micro Pathology	N/A
Treatment	**Appendectomy** with preoperative antibiotic coverage.
Discussion	Peak incidence is in the second and third decades. Causes include **fecaliths** (33%) and **lymphoid hyperplasia** (60%); occasionally caused by tumors (carcinoid tumor is the most common tumor of the appendix), parasites, foreign bodies, and Crohn's disease. Complications include perforation, **periappendiceal abscess,** peritonitis, and generalized or wound sepsis. Differential diagnosis should include enterocolitis, mesenteric lymphadenitis, acute salpingitis, ectopic pregnancy, pain on ovulation (= MITTELSCHMERZ), and Meckel's diverticulum.

APPENDICITIS

ID/CC A **67-year-old** white female complains of increasing fatigue for several months.

HPI She has also noticed significant **weight loss** and **intermittent diarrhea.**

PE Marked **pallor**; palpable left supraclavicular lymph node (= VIRCHOW'S NODE); palpable mass in right iliac fossa; hepatomegaly.

Labs CBC/PBS: microcytic, hypochromic **anemia. Positive stool guaiac test;** elevated serum carcinoembryonic antigen (CEA) levels.

Imaging BE: large, irregular fungating mass in cecum. US: metastatic hepatic nodules. Colonoscopy: large fungating growth in cecum.

Gross Pathology **Cauliflower-like, fungating, nonobstructing growth** in cecum; may be polyploid, sessile, or constricting.

Micro Pathology Well-differentiated adenocarcinoma.

Treatment Right hemicolectomy with temporary colostomy; adjuvant chemotherapy; follow up for recurrence by monitoring CEA levels.

Discussion Early detection by screening for **occult blood in the stool.** The second most common cause of cancer death; incidence increases markedly after age 50. **FIRST AID** p.231

. . . .

CECAL CARCINOMA

ID/CC	A 12-year-old white female, the daughter of **Norwegian** immigrants, complains of **diarrhea and flatulence.**
HPI	Her parents say she has suffered from weight loss despite the fact that she eats well. Her mother adds that her stool is **foul-smelling** and **greasy** (= STEATORRHEA) with no blood or mucus.
PE	Pale and thin; xerosis (= DRYNESS) and hyperkeratosis of skin (due to vitamin A malabsorption); vesicular rash on knees, elbows, and neck; **pruritus with erythematous base** (= DERMATITIS HERPETIFORMIS); cheilosis (= SCALING); ecchymoses (due to vitamin K malabsorption).
Labs	CBC: macrocytic, hypochromic anemia. Lytes: decreased potassium and calcium. Decreased serum cholesterol and albumin; prolonged PT; **abnormal d-xylose test;** positive Sudan stain for fecal fat.
Imaging	UGI/SBFT: loss of mucosal folds and **dilated jejunum.**
Gross Pathology	N/A
Micro Pathology	Hallmark **flattening and atrophy of mucosal villi** with basophilia and loss of nuclear polarity; lymphocytic and plasma cell infiltration of lamina propria.
Treatment	Gluten-free diet.
Discussion	A disease of the small intestine due to **gluten** (gliadin) **hypersensitivity,** it is associated with HLA-DR3 and HLA-DQw2 and is characterized by varying degrees of **nutrient malabsorption:** iron, folate, fat-soluble vitamins (A, D, E, K). Also known as **nontropical sprue** or **celiac sprue.** **FIRST AID** p.237

CELIAC DISEASE

ID/CC   A 45-year-old **alcoholic** male presents with **recurrent epigastric pain** that sometimes radiates to his back.

HPI   He also complains of **bulky, greasy, foul-smelling stool** (= STEATORRHEA). He has lost ten pounds over the past three months.

PE   **Epigastric pain** on deep palpation.

Labs   Quantitative estimation of fat in stool reveals **steatorrhea; elevated serum amylase and lipase levels.**

Imaging   XR-Abdomen: **pancreatic calcification.** CT/US: **pancreatic atrophy and calcification.** ERCP: small stricture of pancreatic duct in head; distal pancreatic duct shows sacculation with intervening **short strictures** (= "CHAIN OF LAKES").

Gross Pathology   **Scarred-down, fibrotic pancreas** with whitish areas of fatty necrosis and areas of cystic cavitation.

Micro Pathology   Pancreatic biopsy reveals presence of dilated ducts, fibrotic stroma, and atrophy of exocrine glands and islets (due to enzymatic fat necrosis).

Treatment   Pancreatic **enzyme replacement; low-fat diet;** surgery for relief of intractable pain.

Discussion   Chronic pancreatitis is a persistent inflammatory disease of the pancreas which is irreversible and causes pain and permanent impairment of endocrine and exocrine function. **Alcohol abuse** is the most common cause in **adults, cystic fibrosis in children.**

. . . .

CHRONIC PANCREATITIS

ID/CC	A 54-year-old white female complains of **colicky pain in the left lower abdomen** and **fever**.
HPI	She has had **frequent attacks of moderate pain** in the same area for several months and one episode of **bloody stools** without excessive mucus.
PE	VS: low-grade fever. PE: pallor; tenderness; rebound and guarding of left lower quadrant but normal stools; **sigmoid colon palpable, thickened, and tender.**
Labs	CBC: **normocytic, normochromic anemia; neutrophilic leukocytosis** with associated left shift (= BANDEMIA). Stool culture reveals no pathogens.
Imaging	CT-Abdomen: diverticular disease with **pericolonic inflammatory stranding.** BE (after acute phase): "saw-toothed" appearance.
Gross Pathology	Resected segment reveals external **outpouchings** up to 1 cm in diameter along colon between tenia coli **from lumen; small mucosal openings lead into pouches.**
Micro Pathology	A diverticulum sectioned along its axis shows **mucosa herniating through a defect in the internal circular layer of muscularis.** Biopsy obtained during sigmoidoscopy reveals no malignancy.
Treatment	**High-fiber diet;** antibiotics for diverticulitis; surgical resection of severely involved segments.
Discussion	A condition of the colon in which the mucosa and submucosa herniate through the muscular layers of the colon to form outpouchings that may become obstructed with feces. Outpouchings may become repeatedly inflamed, resulting in abscess formation, development of fistulas to adjoining organs, colonic obstruction, perforation, and sepsis. Most commonly seen in the **sigmoid colon.** **FIRST AID** p.229

DIVERTICULITIS

ID/CC A 68-year-old black male presents with anorexia, progressive **dysphagia,** odynophagia, and weight loss.

HPI The patient has been drinking very **hot tea** since he was 11 years old and **smokes** one pack of cigarettes per day. His history also reveals heavy **alcohol** intake; occasional cough, vomiting, and **regurgitation;** and severe dysphagia with solids, progressing to liquids.

PE Emaciation; fixed, **nonpainful supraclavicular node;** pale conjunctiva.

Labs CBC/PBS: hypochromic, microcytic anemia. Hemoccult-positive stool; hypoalbuminemia.

Imaging UGI: **irregular fungating esophageal mass** in middle third of esophagus with partial obstruction. CT-Chest: irregular esophageal mass with invasion of mediastinum and enlarged para-aortic lymph node.

Gross Pathology Large fungating mass protruding toward esophageal lumen.

Micro Pathology Squamous cell carcinoma on biopsy.

Treatment Laser ablation of tumor with palliative stent placement; radiotherapy; surgical resection; eventual gastrostomy tube placement.

Discussion The most common variant is **squamous cell carcinoma,** which is associated with alcohol and tobacco use and is more common in blacks. A less common variant is **adenocarcinoma,** which usually involves the distal third of the esophagus and is more common in whites with **Barrett's** (glandular metaplasia of the epithelium of the distal esophagus is caused by chronic, untreated gastroesophageal reflux disease). **FIRST AID** p.231

ESOPHAGEAL CARCINOMA

ID/CC	A 47-year-old white male is brought by ambulance to the emergency room because of **massive, painless vomiting of bright red blood** (= HEMATEMESIS) and shock.
HPI	He is a known homeless **alcoholic** who lives in the streets surrounding the hospital. His friend states that he has been drinking heavily for the past two months.
PE	VS: **tachycardia; hypotension.** PE: skin cold and clammy; **hard nodular hepatomegaly;** mild splenomegaly; spider nevi; caput medusae; clubbing; ascites, mild gynecomastia; bilaterally enlarged parotid glands.
Labs	CBC/PBS: normocytic, normochromic **anemia.** Low serum albumin; **elevated alkaline phosphatase; increased bilirubin, ALT, AST.**
Imaging	EGD: actively bleeding varices.
Gross Pathology	Dilated submucosal esophageal vein secondary to shunting from **portal hypertension;** superficial ulceration, inflammation, and rupture.
Micro Pathology	N/A
Treatment	Restore blood volume, balloon tamponade of varices followed by endoscopic sclerotherapy; splenorenal or other shunt if sclerotherapy fails.
Discussion	Esophageal varices are often silent until they rupture and are associated with a significant mortality rate.

ESOPHAGEAL VARICEAL BLEEDING

ID/CC	A 83-year-old white male complains of **anorexia, frequent vomiting,** and a **gnawing midepigastric pain** of several months' duration.
HPI	The pain is **not relieved by antacids or milk.** The patient has **lost significant weight** over the past few months due to diarrhea after every meal.
PE	Pale, **emaciated** male in moderate distress; left supraclavicular lymph node (= VIRCHOW'S NODE) palpable.
Labs	CBC: **hypochromic, microcytic anemia.** Stool **positive for occult blood;** LFTs normal.
Imaging	UGI: large fungating lesion on greater curvature of stomach with fistulous tract running to transverse colon. EGD: same.
Gross Pathology	Polypoid, raised, fungating mass projecting into lumen; situated at distal end of stomach.
Micro Pathology	Biopsy reveals a **well-differentiated adenocarcinoma** with signet-ring cells.
Treatment	Surgery; radiotherapy; chemotherapy.
Discussion	Chronic atrophic gastritis, pernicious anemia, gastric ulcers, postsurgical gastric remnants, and type A blood are all predisposing risk factors for the development of adenocarcinoma. May spread transperitoneally to the ovaries (= KRUKENBERG TUMOR).

GASTRIC CARCINOMA

ID/CC	A 44-year-old male is admitted to the hospital following episodes of **vomiting blood** (= HEMATEMESIS) and passing **black, tarry, foul-smelling stools** (= MELENA).
HPI	He has experienced **recurrent painless hematemesis** and **melena** for several years, but repeated evaluations have been negative.
PE	Pallor.
Labs	CBC: **microcytic, hypochromic anemia**. Nasogastric aspirate has **coffee-ground** appearance.
Imaging	UGI/EGD: 5-cm mass in fundus of stomach with 2-cm ulcer on surface.
Gross Pathology	Postoperative specimen reveals a firm, circumscribed nodular **mass within the gastric wall** covered by mucosa.
Micro Pathology	Whorling interlaced bundles of spindle-shaped cells; no evidence of anaplasia.
Treatment	Surgical resection.
Discussion	The **most common benign tumor of the stomach.**

Gros

Micro

GASTRIC LEIOMYOMA

ID/CC	A 40-year-old female is admitted to the hospital for evaluation of **neuropsychiatric disturbances, intellectual impairment, and strange movements.**
HPI	She has been diagnosed with **chronic active hepatitis.**
PE	**Icterus; choreiform movements;** slit-lamp examination reveals presence of brownish or gray-green, fine pigmented granules in Descemet's membrane of cornea (= KAYSER–FLEISCHER RING); hepatosplenomegaly.
Labs	**Elevated serum copper; low serum ceruloplasmin; elevated 24-hour urinary copper levels;** LFTs elevated.
Imaging	CT-Head: bilateral hypodensity in basal ganglia.
Gross Pathology	N/A
Micro Pathology	Liver biopsy reveals presence of hepatocellular necrosis in addition to bridging and piecemeal necrosis; Mallory's hyaline seen; liver copper levels elevated.
Treatment	**Penicillamine;** chlorpromazine; liver transplantation.
Discussion	Also known as **hepatolenticular degeneration,** it is an **autosomal-recessive** disorder. The genetic defect is located on chromosome 13, band q14.3. **FIRST AID** p.230

Gros

Micr

ID/CC	A 43-year-old white male complains of severe **burning epigastric pain** and **diarrhea** of two years' duration that has been refractory to medical management.
HPI	The pain awakens him early in the morning, is accompanied by nausea and vomiting, increases with coffee consumption, and also appears 2–3 hours after meals. Three days ago, he also noticed **black stools.**
PE	Slight discomfort on epigastric palpation but no signs of peritoneal irritation; pale skin and mucous membranes; **occult blood** on digital rectal exam.
Labs	Fasting **serum gastrin markedly increased; increased gastric acid output** (= HYPERCHLORHYDRIA) (due to elevated gastrin).
Imaging	CT/MR/Angio: small lesion in pancreas, difficult to localize. UGI/SBFT: atypical ulcers; gastric fold thickening.
Gross Pathology	Ulcers **in uncommon places** in esophagus, duodenum, and jejunum (due to excessive gastrin secretion); **gastrinoma** (commonly in pancreas or duodenum).
Micro Pathology	Usually originate from **delta cells** of pancreas; original lesion may be adenoma, hyperplasia, or carcinoma.
Treatment	High-dose omeprazole; surgical resection if well localized and no metastases; gastrectomy.
Discussion	Causes painful chronic diarrhea (vs. intestinal parasites, carcinoid syndrome, ulcerative colitis); roughly half may be malignant. Associated with **multiple endocrine neoplasia (MEN) type 1** (= WERMER'S SYNDROME).

· ·

ZOLLINGER–ELLISON SYNDROME

ID/CC	An 18-year-old hospitalized male complains of **fever, nausea, vomiting,** and chest pains following a blood transfusion.
HPI	He was involved in a motorcycle accident and was rushed to the emergency room, where he **received five units of blood** before being taken to the OR for repair of a ruptured spleen and liver.
PE	VS: **fever.** PS: no hepatosplenomegaly or lymphadenopathy; surgical laparotomy wound unremarkable.
Labs	**Positive Coombs' test** (indicating autoantibodies to RBCs); decreased serum haptoglobin; elevated indirect bilirubin.
Imaging	N/A
Gross Pathology	N/A
Micro Pathology	N/A
Treatment	Hydration; force diuresis with mannitol or furosemide; hydrocortisone; alkalinize urine with HCO_3.
Discussion	Acute hemolytic transfusion reaction may be the result of complete complement activation; most commonly it is a result of **mismatched blood,** producing **intravascular hemolysis.** If severe, renal shutdown or disseminated intravascular coagulation (DIC) may occur.

. . . .

ACUTE HEMOLYTIC TRANSFUSION REACTION

ID/CC   A 5-year-old white female is brought to her pediatrician because of fever, **marked weakness, pallor, bone pain,** and bleeding from her nose (= EPISTAXIS).

HPI   She has a history of progressively increasing fatigability and **recurrent infections** over the past few months.

PE   VS: fever. PE: marked pallor; epistaxis; ecchymotic patches over skin; **sternal tenderness;** slight hepatosplenomegaly with **nontender lymphadenopathy;** no signs of meningitis; normal funduscopic exam.

Labs   CBC/PBS: normocytic, normochromic **anemia; absolute lymphocytosis with excess blasts (> 30%) and neutropenia; thrombocytopenia.** Common acute lymphoblastic leukemia antigen **(CALLA) (CD10) positive;** terminal deoxytransferase **(TDT) positive** (marker of immature T and B lymphocytes) on enzyme marker studies; negative monospot test for Epstein–Barr virus.

Imaging   CXR: no lymphadenopathy.

Gross Pathology   Neoplastic infiltration of lymph nodes, spleen, liver, and bone marrow with loss of normal architecture.

Micro Pathology   **Myelophthisic bone marrow** (distorted architecture secondary to space-occupying lesions) with lymphoblastic infiltration.

Treatment   Treat infection with antibiotics, **anemia** with blood transfusions, **thrombocytopenia** with platelet concentrations. Remission induction and consolidation chemotherapy. Consider bone marrow transplant.

Discussion   The **most common pediatric neoplasm;** accounts for 80% of all childhood leukemias. Carries a **good prognosis.** **FIRST AID** p.227

· ·

ACUTE LYMPHOBLASTIC LEUKEMIA (ALL)

ID/CC	A **25-year-old woman** presents with **high-grade fever, menorrhagia,** and marked weakness.
HPI	Over the past several weeks, she has also had **recurrent infections.**
PE	Marked **pallor;** multiple purpuric patches over skin; hepatosplenomegaly; **gingival hyperplasia;** sternal tenderness; normal funduscopic and neurologic exam.
Labs	CBC/PBS: normocytic, normochromic **anemia; thrombocytopenia;** leukocytosis composed mainly of **myeloblasts and promyelocytes** (nonmaturing, early blast cells); **neutropenia.** Prolonged PT and PTT.
Imaging	N/A
Gross Pathology	Bone erosion due to **marrow expansion;** chloroma formation, mainly in skull; splenomegaly.
Micro Pathology	Myeloblasts with myelomonocytic differentiation replace normal marrow (= MYELOPHTHISIC BONE MARROW); **basophilic cytoplasmic bodies** (= AUER RODS) in myelocytes; **peroxidase-positive** stains on bone marrow and gingival biopsy.
Treatment	Chemotherapy; bone marrow transplant during first remission if HLA-matched donor available.
Discussion	N/A **FIRST AID** p.227

. . . .

ACUTE MYELOID LEUKEMIA (AML)

ID/CC   A 12-year-old male presents with high fever, marked **pallor**, and **epistaxis**; he has a history of **recurrent URIs** and high-grade fever that have been treated with parenteral antibiotics.

HPI   He has also shown **marked weakness** over the past three months. He lives in the vicinity of an industrial unit that handles petroleum distillates such as **benzene**.

PE   VS: fever. PE: marked pallor of skin and conjunctiva; oral and nasal mucosal **petechiae**; **purpuric patches** visible on skin; no significant lymphadenopathy; no hepatosplenomegaly.

Labs   CBC/PBS: **anemia, neutropenia, and thrombocytopenia** (= PANCYTOPENIA); anemia with low reticulocyte count; normal RBC morphology. Normal serum bilirubin; negative Coombs' test; normal chromosomal studies.

Imaging   N/A

Gross Pathology   Increased yellow marrow and decreased red marrow.

Micro Pathology   Bone marrow nearly acellular and completely fatty; marked decrease in all cell lines.

Treatment   Removal of myelotoxin, in this case benzene; bone marrow transplantation; immunosuppressive treatment; anti-thymocyte globulin; androgens (to stimulate erythropoiesis).

Discussion   Fifty percent of cases are **idiopathic**. Aplastic anemia following **drug or toxin exposure** may be dose dependent (e.g., benzene, cytotoxic drugs) or idiosyncratic (e.g., chloramphenicol). Other causes include **viral infection** and **radiation**. **FIRST AID** p.227

· · · · · · · · · · · · · · · · · · · ·

APLASTIC ANEMIA

ID/CC	A 66-year-old white man recently **diagnosed with chronic lymphocytic leukemia** comes into the emergency room complaining of **fatigue** and tachycardia.
HPI	He also states that his **urine** has been progressively turning **dark and red** over the course of the day.
PE	VS: tachycardia. PE: dyspnea; pallor of skin and mucous membranes; slight jaundice; splenomegaly.
Labs	CBC/PBS: **severe anemia; positive Coombs' test; reticulocytosis;** "bite cells." UA: hemoglobinuria. Increased serum indirect bilirubin.
Imaging	N/A
Gross Pathology	Congestive splenomegaly (due to **extravascular hemolysis** in the spleen).
Micro Pathology	N/A
Treatment	Prednisone; transfusions; splenectomy; immunosuppressive drugs.
Discussion	Idiopathic in about 50% of cases; characterized by autoantibodies against RBC membranes (Rh) and phagocytosis of RBCs by splenic macrophages. Associated with **leukemias, lymphomas,** systemic lupus erythematosus, infections, and drugs (alpha-methyldopa). **FIRST AID** p.227

. . . .

AUTOIMMUNE HEMOLYTIC ANEMIA

ID/CC	A 9-year-old girl, the daughter of **African** immigrants, presents with a large **swelling of the left side her of face and jaw** of **three weeks' duration.**
HPI	Two weeks ago, she complained of **loosening of the** upper second left **molar.** Despite the size of the tumor, there is **no pain** associated with it.
PE	Pallor; large, firm, ill-defined **mass** encompassing entire **upper mandible,** producing mild ipsilateral exophthalmos with **deformation** on left side of face.
Labs	CBC/PBS: normocytic, normochromic anemia; mild leukopenia; positive direct Coombs' test. Karyotype: chromosomal translocation $t(8;14)$ involving c-myc gene.
Imaging	CXR: no evidence of mediastinal widening (vs. Hodgkin's lymphoma).
Gross Pathology	Firm, ill-defined tumor involving upper mandible and deforming neighboring structures, but **no ulceration** or necrosis; **no satellite adenopathy.**
Micro Pathology	Giemsa-stained FNA shows cells of uniform size with nongranular basophilic nuclei and some vacuoles, 2–5 nucleoli, and evenly distributed chromatin surrounded by small, thin, eccentric cytoplasm that is pyroninophilic; high mitotic index and typical "**starry sky**" image pattern.
Treatment	Chemotherapy; alkalinize urine, force diuresis; bone marrow transplantation.
Discussion	A small noncleaved lymphoma (**non-Hodgkin's lymphoma**). Poorly differentiated **B-cell** lymphoblastic lymphoma. The endemic form is characterized by jaw tumors; the nonendemic (Western) form is characterized by abdominal and pelvic involvement. Associated with **Epstein–Barr virus** infections; first described by Denis Burkitt in 1958 in Uganda (endemic in Africa). **FIRST AID** p.227

· · · · · · · · · · · · · · · · · · · ·

BURKITT'S LYMPHOMA

ID/CC	A **65-year-old male** visits his family doctor for a routine annual checkup.
HPI	On directed history, he admits to a **weight loss** of about 12 pounds over the past four months, together with episodes of **epistaxis** and extreme **fatigue**.
PE	Generalized nontender **lymphadenopathy**; pallor; **enlargement of spleen and liver**.
Labs	CBC/PBS: **markedly elevated WBC count** (124,000); **90% lymphocytes**; no lymphoblasts; mild thrombocytopenia; **Coombs-positive hemolytic anemia**; **smudge cells** (fragile lymphocytes).
Imaging	CT/US: hepatosplenomegaly.
Gross Pathology	Lymph node enlargement almost always present; hepatosplenomegaly with tumor nodule formation.
Micro Pathology	Bone marrow biopsy reveals extensive infiltration, mainly by normal-looking lymphocytes and a few lymphoblasts with small, dark, round nuclei and scant cytoplasm; liver, spleen, lymph node involvement common; B-lymphocytes fail to mature properly.
Treatment	Chemotherapy; prednisone; splenectomy.
Discussion	A malignant neoplastic disease of **B lymphocytes**; characterized by slow progression of anemia, hemolytic anemia, recurrent infections, lymph node enlargement, and bleeding episodes. **FIRST AID** p.227

ID/CC	A 55-year-old white male visits a doctor for a life insurance physical examination.
HPI	The patient has no major complaints except for occasional **fatigue** and **increasing abdominal girth**.
PE	Pallor of skin and mucous membranes; **markedly enlarged spleen; pain on palpation over sternum;** no lymphadenopathy; no other abnormalities found.
Labs	CBC/PBS: **markedly elevated WBC count** (130,000); immature granulocytes mixed with normal-appearing ones; **basophilia;** early thrombocytosis; late thrombocytopenia. **Low leukocyte alkaline phosphatase;** elevated serum vitamin B$_{12}$ level. Karyotype: chromosomal translocation **t(9;22)** (= PHILADELPHIA CHROMOSOME).
Imaging	US-Abdomen: splenomegaly.
Gross Pathology	Skull chloromas (malignant, green-colored tumor arising from myeloid tissue); enlarged and congested spleen with areas of thrombosis and microinfarcts; hepatomegaly (due to proliferation and infiltration by granulocyte precursors and mature granulocytes).
Micro Pathology	Hepatic sinusoidal leukemic infiltrates; congestive splenomegaly with myeloid metaplasia; Philadelphia chromosome in all myeloid progeny.
Treatment	Hydroxyurea; alpha-interferon; leukapheresis; bone marrow transplantation. Treatment ineffective after development of blast crisis.
Discussion	Death usually results from accelerated transformation into acute leukemia (= BLAST CRISIS) within 2–5 years. **FIRST AID** p.227

. . . .

CHRONIC MYELOGENOUS LEUKEMIA (CML)

ID/CC	A 25-year-old white female **continues to bleed** steadily after a normal, spontaneous vaginal delivery.
HPI	Manual exploration of the uterus reveals retained placental tissue that requires dilatation and curettage; 30 minutes after the procedure, the patient begins to **bleed profusely from her gums** and continues to bleed vaginally.
PE	Diffuse bleeding in gums and oral mucosa; **bleeding diathesis of skin** (both petechiae and purpura) with **oozing from venipuncture sites**.
Labs	Low fibrinogen. CBC: low platelet count. Prolonged PT and activated PTT; elevated fibrin split products.
Imaging	N/A
Gross Pathology	May see complications such as renal cortical necrosis, limb thrombosis with gangrene, and ischemic adrenal necrosis.
Micro Pathology	Microthrombi in arterioles and capillaries, leading to **microinfarcts** in practically any organ; also **hemorrhages** and petechiae in involved organs.
Treatment	Treat underlying disorder; fresh frozen plasma; fibrinogen cryoprecipitate; platelets; aminocaproic acid with heparin.
Discussion	A bleeding disorder due to depletion of platelets and coagulation factors secondary to excessive clotting in microcirculation. Precipitated by **cancer, septicemia, burns,** multiple **trauma,** and **obstetric complications.**

· ·

DISSEMINATED INTRAVASCULAR COAGULATION (DIC)

ID/CC	**During the administration of a blood transfusion,** a 45-year-old male presents with **fever, headache, and facial flushing.**
HPI	An hour later he develops **frank rigors.** He has received **several transfusions in the past,** all of which were uneventful. The last one was **a few weeks ago.**
PE	VS: fever; normotension; tachycardia. PE: marked pallor; facial flushing; no cyanosis, icterus, or respiratory distress evident.
Labs	CBC/PBS: **negative direct and indirect Coombs' test.** Normal serum bilirubin; no incompatibility found on repeat cross-matching of donor serum and patient's blood.
Imaging	N/A
Gross Pathology	N/A
Micro Pathology	N/A
Treatment	Supportive; antipyretics; **leukocyte-deplete future transfusions** by filtration.
Discussion	Caused by **preformed leukoagglutinins** (cytotoxic antibodies) developed after previous transfusion; primarily a **type II hypersensitivity reaction.** Skin rash and pruritus or anaphylaxis occur in allergic reactions mediated by IgE (due to a **type 1 hypersensitivity reaction**).

· ·

FEBRILE NONHEMOLYTIC TRANSFUSION REACTION

ID/CC	A 45-year-old male with refractory acute myeloid leukemia is brought to the emergency room with **fever**, a **generalized rash, jaundice,** right upper quadrant pain, severe **diarrhea,** and dyspnea.
HPI	Two months ago, he underwent an apparently uncomplicated **bone marrow transplantation.** Prior to the transplant, he received total body irradiation, chemotherapy, and broad-spectrum antibiotics.
PE	VS: normotension. PE: cachexia; moderate dehydration; jaundice; **violaceous and erythematous macules, papules, bullae,** and scale formation over extremities.
Labs	**Elevated IgE level.** CBC/PBS: falling blood counts (WBCs, hematocrit, and platelets); relative eosinophilia. Elevated direct serum bilirubin and transaminases; no infectious agents on stool exam.
Imaging	N/A
Gross Pathology	Destruction of intestinal mucosa, liver, and skin; interstitial pneumonia.
Micro Pathology	Vacuolar changes of basal cell layer on skin biopsy with perivenular lymphocytic infiltrates (**CD8+ T cells**).
Treatment	Cyclosporin A, alone or with methotrexate, rabbit antihuman thymocyte globulin (ATG), methyl-prednisolone or anti-T-cell monoclonal antibodies.
Discussion	Donor lymphocytes can produce GVHD in immunosuppressed recipients. Occurs in one-third of bone marrow transplant recipients.

. . . .

GRAFT-VERSUS-HOST DISEASE (GVHD)

ID/CC	A 61-year-old **male** presents with marked **weakness, gingival bleeding,** and an **abdominal mass.**
HPI	He has a history of **recurrent bacterial infections** and has not traveled outside the U.S.
PE	**Pallor; marked splenomegaly;** mild hepatomegaly; no lymphadenopathy, icterus, or ascites.
Labs	CBC/PBS: **anemia; decreased WBCs and platelets** (= PANCYTOPENIA); **leukocytes with characteristic long, thin cytoplasmic projections** (= "HAIRY CELLS").
Imaging	CXR: normal. CT/US-Abdomen: massive splenomegaly; mild hepatomegaly; no lymphadenopathy; no evidence of portal hypertension.
Gross Pathology	Liver, spleen, and bone marrow infiltrated by leukemic cells; splenomegaly may be significant.
Micro Pathology	**Bone marrow largely replaced by leukemic cells** (= MYELOPHTHISIC BONE MARROW); large proportion are hairy cells and contain tartrate-resistant acid phosphatase (**TRAP**); splenic biopsy reveals leukemic infiltration of red pulp by hairy cells.
Treatment	Pentostatin (80% remission rate); splenectomy; alpha-interferon.
Discussion	Chronic B-cell malignancy; autoimmune syndromes are frequently seen, including vasculitis and arthritis; **atypical mycobacterial infections.**

· ·

HAIRY CELL LEUKEMIA

ID/CC   A **1-year-old** white **girl** is brought into the emergency room because of sudden weakness, apathy, **easy bruisability,** and **periorbital edema with low urinary volumes.**

HPI   The infant experienced **diarrhea** and had vomited for two days, but her condition **resolved spontaneously** four days before admission.

PE   Pallor; listlessness; hepatomegaly; ankle and **periorbital edema; purpuric rash** on chest and limbs.

Labs   CBC/PBS: severe **anemia; low platelet count; RBC fragmentation** (burr-shaped erythrocytes); negative Coombs' test. UA: proteinuria; hematuria; **RBC casts.** Markedly **increased LDH;** normal coagulation profile.

Imaging   N/A

Gross Pathology   Ischemic renal cortical necrosis.

Micro Pathology   Focal glomerular necrosis with capillary endothelial hyaline thrombi.

Treatment   Conservative management of acute renal failure (in children); plasmapheresis (in adults).

Discussion   Acute renal failure and microangiopathic hemolytic anemia occurring after bacterial (enterohemorrhagic *E. coli, Shigella*) or viral infection; a **common cause of acute renal failure in children.**

HEMOLYTIC–UREMIC SYNDROME

ID/CC	An **8-year-old** white male presents with an erythematous skin **rash over the buttocks and legs** coupled with **joint pains** and **hematuria.**
HPI	Three days before he had complained of cough, coryza, low-grade fever, and sore throat. He has a **history of allergy** to dust and pollen.
PE	VS: hypertension. PE: **palpable purpuric skin lesions** over buttocks and legs; painful restriction of knee and ankle joint movement with swelling.
Labs	CBC: **normal platelet count;** normal coagulation tests. Increased ESR; increased BUN and serum creatinine. UA: **RBCs and RBC casts** on urinary sediment. Positive stool guaiac test (due to occult blood).
Imaging	N/A
Gross Pathology	Necrotizing vasculitis of kidneys and lungs.
Micro Pathology	Renal biopsy shows focal and segmental glomerulonephritis with crescents (mesangioproliferative); **mesangial IgA deposits** on immunofluorescence.
Treatment	Supportive; steroids; high-dose immunoglobulin therapy experimental.
Discussion	An idiopathic disorder also known as anaphylactoid or vascular purpura; **common vasculitis in children.**

HENOCH–SCHÖNLEIN PURPURA

ID/CC   A **24-year-old** white male complains of rapid enlargement of his abdomen, producing a dragging sensation, along with a **painless lump in his neck** for the past two months.

HPI   The patient also complains of intermittent **fever**, drenching **night sweats**, pruritus, and **significant weight loss.**

PE   Pallor; **unilateral nontender, rubbery, enlarged cervical lymph nodes; splenomegaly;** no enlargement of tonsils.

Labs   CBC/PBS: neutrophilic leukocytosis with lymphopenia; normocytic anemia. Elevated ESR; elevated serum copper and ferritin; negative Mantoux test.

Imaging   CXR: **bilateral hilar lymphadenopathy.**

Gross Pathology   Involved lymph nodes are rubbery and have **"cut-potato"** appearance of cut surface.

Micro Pathology   Lymph node biopsy shows large histiocyte cells with multilobed nuclei and eosinophilic nucleolus resembling **owl's eyes** (= REED–STERNBERG CELLS); no bone marrow involvement on bone marrow biopsy.

Treatment   Radiotherapy and chemotherapy.

Discussion   Four patterns of Hodgkin's disease are seen on lymph node biopsy: lymphocytic predominance 10%–20%; nodular sclerosis 40%–60% (seen frequently in young women); mixed cellularity 20%–40%; and lymphocyte depleted 10%. Prognosis worsens in this order. **Ann Arbor staging:** I–IV with subclassification A (no constitutional symptoms) and B (weight loss, fever, night sweats).

· ·

HODGKIN'S LYMPHOMA

ID/CC	A **3-year-old** white female is brought to the emergency room with a skin rash and **severe epistaxis.**
HPI	The patient had a **URI** consisting of a severe cough and a runny nose five days **before the onset of her symptoms.** She has a history of **prolonged bleeding** following minimal trauma; her father has been diagnosed with a bleeding disorder.
PE	**Mucosal petechiae;** epistaxis; **hemorrhagic bullae** in buccal mucosa.
Labs	CBC: mild anemia; **low platelet count** (10,000); **RBCs and WBCs normal.** Prolonged bleeding time; normal PTT; normal PT.
Imaging	N/A
Gross Pathology	**Purpura** (due to extravasation of blood from intravascular space into skin); pin-sized hemorrhages (= PETECHIAE); ecchymosis (larger than petechiae but smaller than purpura).
Micro Pathology	Normal bone marrow aspirate with **increased number of megakaryocytes.**
Treatment	Prednisone; splenectomy; danazol.
Discussion	An **autoimmune** disease with formation of IgG anti-platelet antibodies and subsequent platelet destruction in the spleen.

IDIOPATHIC THROMBOCYTOPENIC PURPURA (ITP)

ID/CC	A **64-year-old** black male suffers from **bone pain**, weight loss, and **easy fatigability**.
HPI	He also complains of **recurrent URIs**.
PE	Pallor; **bone tenderness**; petechiae on buccal mucosa; no hepatosplenomegaly.
Labs	CBC/PBS: **normocytic, normochromic anemia**; neutropenia; **rouleau formation** (RBCs adhering together like stack of poker chips). **Elevated serum calcium**; normal alkaline phosphatase; markedly **increased ESR; gamma spike on serum protein electrophoresis** (monoclonal gammopathy). UA: **Bence Jones proteinuria** (due to IgG light chains).
Imaging	XR-Plain: **punched-out, lytic bone lesions** in vertebrae, long bones, and skull (axial skeleton).
Gross Pathology	Multifocal replacement of normal bone tissue with tumor cells (plasmacytoma); pelvis, skull, and spine most affected.
Micro Pathology	Infiltration of bone marrow by normal-looking plasma cells (abundant cytoplasm, eccentric nuclei) in aggregates; **amyloid deposits** in kidney with renal tubular cast formation and interstitial fibrosis (can cause **renal insufficiency**); bone erosion and destruction of cortical bone.
Treatment	Various combinations of alkylating agents.
Discussion	A **primary malignancy of plasma cells** with replacement of normal bone marrow; the most common primary bone cancer. **FIRST AID** p.227

· ·

MULTIPLE MYELOMA

ID/CC	A 54-year-old white male complains of **easy fatigability,** shortness of breath, headache, and lightheadedness over the course of almost one year, with increasing severity.
HPI	He has also noticed a feeling of heaviness in his abdomen and **increasing girth** as well as recurrent deep pain in the legs and occasionally in the upper abdomen.
PE	**Massive splenomegaly;** enlarged liver; moderate amount of ascitic fluid; multiple petechiae on thorax and extremities; **no lymphadenopathy** (one differential feature shared with chronic myelogenous leukemia).
Labs	CBC/PBS: anemia (Hb 7.2); **low hematocrit;** anemia; immature WBCs and normoblasts seen simultaneously (= LEUKOERYTHROBLASTIC SMEAR); **teardrop-shaped RBCs.**
Imaging	XR-Plain: dense bones (generalized osteosclerosis).
Gross Pathology	**Extramedullary hematopoiesis,** which is prominent in liver and spleen, with significant increase in size and weight together with firm consistency.
Micro Pathology	**"Dry tap"** on **bone marrow** biopsy; hypocellular bone marrow (hypercellular early in disease); significant increase in number of megakaryocytes; replacement of marrow tissue with fibrosis (positive reticulin on silver stain); preservation of normal architecture of spleen.
Treatment	Transfusions; androgens; alpha-interferon; splenectomy.
Discussion	Also called agnogenic myeloid metaplasia, it is idiopathic. Increased secretion of platelet-derived growth factor (PDGF) causes **replacement of bone marrow tissue with fibrosis.**

MYELOFIBROSIS WITH MYELOID METAPLASIA

ID/CC	A 53-year-old white male notices **painless lumps** bilaterally **in his neck** that have slowly enlarged over the past three months.
HPI	Although he denies any pain, he admits to having episodes of mild **fever, night sweats,** and some **weight loss** over this period.
PE	Bilateral cervical **firm lymphadenopathy;** pallor; splenomegaly.
Labs	CBC: Coombs-positive hemolytic **anemia;** thrombocytopenia. **Elevated serum LDH;** hypogammaglobulinemia.
Imaging	CT/US: lymphadenopathy; splenomegaly.
Gross Pathology	Lymph nodes have grayish hue on outside and **"cut-potato"** appearance of cut surface.
Micro Pathology	Lymph node biopsy demonstrates nodular (well-differentiated) or diffuse type (poorly differentiated) lymphocytic lymphoma; histiocytic and stem cell lymphoma.
Treatment	Alkylating agents in various combinations; radiotherapy if localized; bone marrow transplantation.
Discussion	Primary malignant neoplasms of lymphocytes arise in lymphoid tissue anywhere in the body; mainly in lymph nodes, but may involve intra-abdominal organs and bone marrow.

ID/CC	A **12-year-old male** presents with a **swelling** above the right knee and associated pain.
HPI	There is **no history of trauma** at the site of pain. There has been **no discharge** from the swollen region and **no fever**.
PE	**Bony-hard**, tender, roughly circular swelling above right knee (**distal femur**); overlying skin temperature normal; mechanical restriction of movement of right knee.
Labs	Normal ESR; **elevated serum alkaline phosphatase** (may be used as marker of treatment response).
Imaging	XR-Plain: osteoblastic bone lesion at distal end of femur with characteristic **"sunburst" or "onion-peel"** periosteal reaction; periosteal elevation by metaphyseal tumor (= CODMAN'S TRIANGLE).
Gross Pathology	Firm, whitish mass with **osteoblastic** bone sclerosis originating from metaphysis adjacent to epiphyseal growth plate and invading through cortex, lifting up periosteum.
Micro Pathology	Bone biopsy shows multinucleated giant cells, anaplastic cells with pleomorphism, and osteoid production with foci of sarcomatous degeneration.
Treatment	Surgical amputation; consider limb salvage; radiotherapy, chemotherapy.
Discussion	A primary malignant tumor of bone, it may be osteoblastic or osteolytic. Pathologic fractures may occur; pulmonary metastases are frequent.

OSTEOGENIC SARCOMA

ID/CC	A 62-year-old **Jewish** male visits his family doctor because of **epistaxis**, headache, and dizziness.
HPI	The patient had **black, tarry stools** (= MELENA) two months ago and was previously admitted to the hospital for **deep venous thrombosis.** He also describes episodes of severe generalized **itching** (= PRURITUS), primarily after showering.
PE	VS: **hypertension** (BP 170/100). PE: obese and **plethoric;** mild cyanosis; engorged, tortuous retinal veins with dark red hue on funduscopy; palpable **spleen.**
Labs	CBC: **markedly increased RBC count;** WBCs and platelets also increased. Normal PO_2, PCO_2, and PT; increased vitamin B_{12} levels; increased leukocyte alkaline phosphatase; increased serum and urine uric acid levels; **decreased erythropoietin level.**
Imaging	N/A
Gross Pathology	**Increased blood volume and viscosity** (RBC **sludging** and thrombus formation mainly in heart and brain); subnormal platelet function (bleeding tendency); increased frequency of peptic ulceration.
Micro Pathology	Bone marrow biopsy shows **increase in erythroid series precursors** and, to a lesser extent, in megakaryocytes and WBC precursors; thrombus formation with microinfarcts in brain and heart; myelofibrosis may ensue with characteristic findings.
Treatment	Phlebotomy; hydroxyurea; alpha-interferon; treat hyperuricemia.
Discussion	An increase in RBC mass with increased blood volume and viscosity; may be primary (polycythemia rubra vera) or secondary (due to COPD, smoking, obesity, etc.). It may progress to chronic myelogenous leukemia or acute myelogenous leukemia.

POLYCYTHEMIA VERA (PCV)

ID/CC	An **18-month-old boy** presents with **diminished visual acuity** and a wandering right eye that his mother noticed while watching him play with his toys.
HPI	On directed history, the child admits to having **eye pain** at night.
PE	**White amaurotic "cat's eye" reflex** in right eye; deviation of right eye (= STRABISMUS); **tenderness in eye** on gentle compression; **intraocular mass** on retinal examination.
Labs	N/A
Imaging	CT/MR-Orbit: lobulated, hyperdense retrolental (behind lens) mass; no optic nerve compression.
Gross Pathology	Whitish mass behind lens.
Micro Pathology	Sheets of small, round blue cells with clusters of cuboidal or short columnar cells arranged around a central lumen (= FLEXNER–WINTERSTEINER ROSETTES).
Treatment	Surgery.
Discussion	The **nonhereditary** variety appear as a single tumor; **hereditary** forms occur in early childhood and are often bilateral or multicentric. Cytogenetic studies reveal a **deletion on chromosome 13** (band 14 on long arm, Rb gene).

ID/CC	A term female newborn is noted to have **edema, dyspnea, cyanosis, and marked jaundice.**
HPI	Her **mother is blood type AB Rh-negative.** Her **previous childbirth** was an uneventful full-term vaginal delivery conducted outside the United States four years ago. The mother **did not receive any subsequent immunizations.**
PE	Pallor; **marked jaundice;** hypotonia; S3 and S4; hepatosplenomegaly; **generalized edema.**
Labs	Blood type of **mother AB Rh negative;** blood type of father A Rh positive; **blood type of first child** A **Rh positive.** Mother's serum: **positive** indirect **Coombs' test,** anti-D antibody titer > 1:64. Neonate's serum: positive direct Coombs' test, increased indirect bilirubin.
Imaging	N/A
Gross Pathology	Brain specimen from autopsy reveals yellow staining of basal ganglia by unconjugated bilirubin (= KERNICTERUS).
Micro Pathology	N/A
Treatment	Phototherapy (promotes elimination of bilirubin); exchange transfusion.
Discussion	The mother produced anti-D (IgG) antibodies due to her exposure to D antigen during her delivery of Rh-positive infant. In her subsequent pregnancy, these antibodies reacted with the fetus's RBCs (Rh positive), producing hemolysis and **fetal heart failure with generalized edema** (= HYDROPS FETALIS). To prevent Rh isoimmunization, all Rh-negative mothers with an Rh-positive fetus should receive **RhO (D) immune globulin** following deliveries, abortions, ectopic pregnancies, or even amniocentesis.

. . . .

RH HEMOLYTIC DISEASE OF NEWBORN

ID/CC	A 4-year-old female is brought by her mother to the pediatric clinic after she finds **blood and a "lump" in the child's vagina.**
HPI	The child's father died of brain cancer, and her mother is receiving treatment for breast cancer. Her grandfather died of metastatic colorectal cancer.
PE	Pelvic exam reveals **ulcerated, polypoid, grape-like mass** arising from wall of vagina.
Labs	Routine lab work on urine, blood, and stool yields no pathologic findings.
Imaging	N/A
Gross Pathology	Bulky tumor mass with multilobed papillary projections resembling mass of grapes.
Micro Pathology	Biopsy of tumor mass shows **desmin- and myoglobin-positive** (muscle tumor), elongated rhabdomyoblasts with large eosinophilic cytoplasm and **cross-striations.**
Treatment	Surgical resection with adjuvant chemotherapy, radiotherapy.
Discussion	A subtype of **embryonal rhabdomyosarcoma** that characteristically protrudes like a mass of grapes from the vagina or bladder, it is the most common sarcoma in children. Rhabdomyosarcomas are often found in **"cancer families"** (e.g., Li–Fraumeni syndrome).

. . . .

SARCOMA BOTRYOIDES

ID/CC	A 6-year-old white female is brought to the emergency room by her mother because of severe **itching, joint pain,** and a **generalized skin eruption.**
HPI	She had received an **injection of penicillin six days before** for streptococcal tonsillitis. Her mother denies any relevant past medical history, including allergies. Once in the hospital, the child developed fever, **edema** of the ankles and knees, hematuria, and lethargy.
PE	Generalized **urticarial skin rash;** axillary and inguinal lymphadenopathy; splenomegaly; redness and swelling of knees and ankles.
Labs	UA: proteinuria; hematuria.
Imaging	N/A
Gross Pathology	Generalized wheals throughout body.
Micro Pathology	Vascular lesions show fibrinoid necrosis and a neutrophilic infiltrate; **immune complex deposition in kidney and joints.**
Treatment	Epinephrine if severe; antihistamines; corticosteroids.
Discussion	**Type III hypersensitivity reaction** (immune complex disease) with a latency period between exposure to the offending agent (drugs, serum) and the appearance of signs and symptoms; usually self-limiting. **FIRST AID** p.208

. . . .

SERUM SICKNESS

ID/CC A 23-year-old white **female** diagnosed two years ago as **HIV positive** is brought to the emergency room by her husband because of tachycardia, shortness of breath, headache, **intermittent disorientation**, and aphasia.

HPI She had started prophylactic **SMX–TMP** three weeks ago. On the previous day, she had finished her menstrual period, which was abundant and had lasted for seven days. Her husband also points out a **generalized red rash** all over her body.

PE VS: tachycardia; **fever**. PE: pale skin and mucous membranes; **confusion** and apathy **with lucid periods**; **petechiae** on chest and extremities; positive Babinski's sign.

Labs CBC/PBS: microangiopathic hemolytic anemia (Hb 7.2) with striking **reticulocytosis** and **damaged RBCs** (= SCHISTOCYTES); **low platelet count** (50,000); negative Coombs' test. Elevated indirect bilirubin (3.5). UA: hematuria. **Absent haptoglobin** (due to intravascular hemolysis); **normal coagulation tests.**

Imaging N/A

Gross Pathology Thrombus formation in several organs with platelet depletion and microangiopathic hemolytic anemia; kidney, brain, and heart most affected by thrombosis.

Micro Pathology Multiple hyaline thrombi in brain, myocardium, renal cortex, adrenals, and pancreas.

Treatment Plasmapheresis and fresh frozen plasma exchange; prednisone; splenectomy.

Discussion Also known as Moschcowitz's syndrome, it is an idiopathic disease found in **pregnant** and **HIV-positive** patients and following exposure to drugs such as **antibiotics** and **estrogens.**

THROMBOTIC THROMBOCYTOPENIC PURPURA (TTP)

ID/CC	A 12-year-old white female is brought to the emergency room because of **uncontrollable bleeding following a tooth extraction.**
HPI	She has a **history of prolonged bleeding** following minimal trauma. Her **father** also has a **bleeding disorder.**
PE	Mucosal petechiae; epistaxis.
Labs	**Prolonged bleeding time; moderately prolonged PTT; quantitative assay for factor VIII reduced;** platelets do not aggregate with ristocetin test; low von Willebrand's factor (vWF) antigen levels; low vWF activity.
Imaging	N/A
Gross Pathology	N/A
Micro Pathology	N/A
Treatment	Desmopressin, virally attenuated vWF concentrate (Humate-P); avoid aspirin.
Discussion	A common congenital disorder of hemostasis; also called vascular hemophilia. Types I and II are **autosomal dominant;** vWF factor is necessary for platelet adhesion.

· ·

VON WILLEBRAND'S DISEASE

ID/CC	A **68-year-old** white male visits his doctor complaining of **weight loss,** increasing **fatigue, weakness,** headache, and **visual disturbances** over the past several months.
HPI	He also complains of **easy bruising** and **bleeding gums** while brushing his teeth.
PE	Generalized **lymphadenopathy; engorgement of retinal veins** with hemorrhages; moderate hepatosplenomegaly.
Labs	CBC/PBS: anemia (Hb 7.3); RBC **rouleau formation. IgM paraprotein** (monoclonal spike on serum protein electrophoresis); increased scrum viscosity.
Imaging	XR-Plain: **absence of lytic lesions** (vs. multiple myeloma).
Gross Pathology	N/A
Micro Pathology	Lymph node biopsy may be labeled pleomorphic lymphoma; bone marrow and spleen typically infiltrated with plasma cell precursors (plasmacytic lymphocytes); may show cytoplasmic eosinophilic, PAS-positive inclusion bodies (= DUTCHER BODIES).
Treatment	Plasmapheresis; chlorambucil; cyclophosphamide.
Discussion	A B-lymphocyte disorder characterized by **excessive IgM** (macroglobulin) **production** and **hyperviscosity syndrome.**

. . . .

WALDENSTRÖM'S MACROGLOBULINEMIA

ID/CC	A 2-year-old **male** is brought to his pediatrician because of recurrent **epistaxis** and chronic **eczematous dermatitis**.
HPI	He has a history of **recurring pneumonia** and bilateral **chronic** suppurative **otitis media**. A **male cousin** suffers from a **similar illness**.
PE	Epistaxis; eczematous dermatitis over both legs; several **purpuric patches** over skin; mild splenomegaly and cervical lymphadenopathy.
Labs	CBC/PBS: **thrombocytopenia;** lymphopenia. Decreased isohemagglutinins; decreased IgM; increased IgE, IgG, and IgA; **inability to form antibody to carbohydrate antigens.**
Imaging	N/A
Gross Pathology	N/A
Micro Pathology	N/A
Treatment	Largely supportive; bone marrow transplant; splenectomy.
Discussion	An **X-linked recessive** disease characterized by a **triad of thrombocytopenia, eczema, and recurrent infections,** it is due to a deletion of the WASP gene in the p11 region of the X chromosome. Associated with an increased incidence of **lymphomas.**

. . . .

WISKOTT–ALDRICH SYNDROME

From the authors of *Underground Clinical Vignettes*

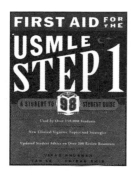

A true classic used by over 200,000 students around the world. The '99 edition features details on the new computerized test, new color plates and thoroughly updated high-yield facts and book reviews. Bi-directional links with the *Underground Clinical Vignettes Step 1* series. ISBN 0-8385-2612-8.

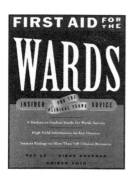

This high-yield student-to-student guide is designed to help students make the transition from the basic sciences to the hospital wards and succeed on their clinical rotations. The book features an orientation to the hospital environment, tips on being an effective and efficient junior medical student, student-proven advice tailored to each core rotation, a database of high-yield clinical facts, and recommendations for clinical pocket books, texts, and references. ISBN 0-8385-2595-4.

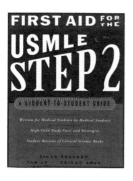

This entirely rewritten second edition now follows in the footsteps of *First Aid for the USMLE Step 1*. Features an exam preparation guide geared to the new computerized test, basic science and clinical high-yield facts, color plates and ratings of USMLE Step 2 books and software. Bi-directional links with the *Underground Clinical Vignettes Step 2* series.

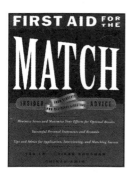

This top rated (5 stars, *Doody Review*) student-to-student guide helps medical students effectively and efficiently navigate the residency application process, helping them make the most of their limited time, money, and energy. The book draws on the advice and experiences of successful student applicants as well as residency directors. Also featured are application and interview tips tailored to each specialty, successful personal statements and CVs with analyses, current trends, and common interview questions with suggested strategies for responding. ISBN 0-8385-2596-2.

The *First Aid* series by Appleton & Lange...the review book leader.
Available through your local health sciences bookstore !

About the Authors

....

VIKAS BHUSHAN, MD
Vikas is a diagnostic radiologist in Los Angeles and the series editor for *Underground Clinical Vignettes*. His intcrests include traveling, reading, writing, and world music. He is single and can be reached at vbhushan@aol.com

CHIRAG AMIN, MD
Chirag is an orthopedics resident at Orlando Regional Medical Center. He plans on pursuing a spine fellowship. He can be reached at chiragamin@aol.com

TAO LE, MD
Tao is completing a medicine residency at Yale-New Haven Hospital and is applying for a fellowship in allergy and immunology. He is married to Thao, who is a pediatrics resident. He can be reached at taotle@aol.com

VISHAL PALL, MBBS
Vishal recently completed medical school and internship in Chandigarh, India. He hopes to begin his Internal Medicine residency training in the US in July 1999. He can be reached at vishalpall@hotmail.com

HOANG NGUYEN
Hoang (Henry) is a third-year medical student at Northwestern University. Henry is single and lives in Chicago, where he spends his free time writing, reading, and enjoying music. He can be reached at hbnguyen@nwu.edu

JOSE M. FIERRO, MD
Jose (Pepe) is beginning a med/peds residency at Brookdale University Hospital in New York. He was a general surgeon in Mexico and worked extensively in Central Africa. His interests include world citizenship and ethnic music. He is married and can be reached at jmfierro@aol.com

VIPAL SONI
Vipal (Vip) is a fourth-year medical student at the UCLA School of Medicine. His interests include music and tennis. Vip is single and lives in Los Angeles. He can be reached at vsoni@ucla.edu